"Revealing My Depression Treatment"

A Memoir

Contains The Wisdom of
Psychotherapists as experienced
by the patient "*Bud*" David Bozyk

Table of Contents

Acknowledgements

1. One Dr. R. explained to me that it would be best not to include names of contributing psychotherapists in this script. Reason: to avoid any possible legal complications, e.g. see example under Preface.

2. Another psychotherapist suggested that I include the name of Dr. Michael Yapko, world renowned for the treatment of depression.

3. One of my very well qualified psychotherapists has read all of this book's contents and has approved of same.

Sincerely,

David B. Bozyk

Preface

Dear Reader:

Dr. J.F.T. Young, a professor of physics at the University of Manitoba once said to our class, "*Science moves forward on crutches.*" I intended to complete this writing long ago, and now feel that my progress in writing it has moved forward on "*broken crutches!*"

When I was four years old I was the only family member who could not read. I asked our mother if I could be taught how to read, her reply: "*You will be taught how to read when you start to go to school.*" With that reply I felt depressed, went back to our bookcase resulting in failed attempts to learn how to read on my own.

When I started school I felt alone and frightened. I cried so often that I failed the first grade and for years felt ashamed.

At age fifteen I went to see our family physician, to have him refer me to a psychotherapist. He told me that the fee was $10.00, a price that our family could not afford.

Years later I sought help from several psychotherapists. Included in this script is information from these psychotherapists which may be beneficial to the reader.

In order to avoid any possible legal repercussions, I have excluded names and any linkage to ALL psychotherapists I have seen. Reason: see Vancouver Sun Jan. 6, 2015. "*North Shore psychiatrist voluntarily surrenders licence for ...*". However, I have name one psychotherapist who is recognized as a world renowned specialist on depression. Please see end of Chapter 15.

The purpose of the information gathered herein, is to share its benefits for people suffering from depression and anxiety. For example: psychological explanations of older family members and their *"pecking order attitudes"* towards their younger siblings.

After three years, one psychotherapist asked me if I had seen improvement in myself. My reply was, *"To tell you the truth I do not."* This psychotherapist gave me his negative appraisal which would likely have a detrimental impact even on someone who was NOT depressed. This psychotheraPIST ME OFF by saying to me, *"HERE IS NO HOPE!"*

The effects of my early childhood experiences remind me of what the poet Alexander Pope wrote, *"Tis education forms the common mind; Just as the twig is bent the tree's inclined."*

When I attended the Seniors' Depression Support Group in North Vancouver, unlike most members, because of my feelings of inferiority, poverty, fear, and shame, I could not speak about myself and my family experiences. Therefore, I asked if it would be acceptable for me to write about my background for other members to read. This method was accepted. And because of his very tragic experiences, I said that I would address some of my revelations to a member named "Stan" – all members agreed.

Many people believe that the last born child in the family is *"spoiled."* I was the last born of five children and this is a concise preview of some of my upbringing:

- I was told that I was too slow. I remember listening to our mother explaining to visiting relatives that I was as slow as one uncle who was slow in speech and movements.

- I was often criticized for my behaviour. e.g. Adam, a family friend once asked me, *"Why do your brothers talk about you that way?"* My reply *"I don't know."* Adam answered, *"They want to put you down, suppress you!"*

- While still a preschooler, and for over ten years thereafter, I was teased* and laughed at** by my mother and older sister because one of my playmates was a girl! When they mentioned this girl's name with a smile, I would walk away in shame.

---

* *"Teasing can easily reach to the level of being considered bullying. Teasing is a negative behaviour directed at a weaker, smaller, often different sort of person than the bully, and often escalates"* From: wikianswers.com

***"Laughter... for some, the mere sight of a smile or hearing laughter, is enough to elicit shame, anxiety, and fear in general, originates from repeated experiences of being ridiculed or put down during childhood and adolescence."* From: T. Platt, Department of Psych. U. of Zurich, Switzerland

I began continued treatment for my depression when I was 50 years old, which lasted through age 90, i.e. 40 years.

Sincerely,

David *"Bud"* Bozyk

Chapter 1 - Fear of my Father's voice!

The following are the verbal instructions of a psychotherapist, with me going into a hypnotic state. You might feel a hypnotic effect if you read it slowly. The topic is my fear of my father's loud voice. My father was a corporal in the peacetime Austrian army.

Psychotherapist:

Okay, Bud, a chance to do some hypnosis.

And think about the impact of your dad, the corporal and his corporal voice, and how frightening that would be to a kid. There are a lot of stories in movies about army, navy, and air force fathers coming home and lording it over their kids like they were lorded over. And it's a form of cheap power in the sense that he is using army tactics within the family, which are not appropriate—because it frightens people. A loving father does not want to frighten his children.

So he made a mistake and it had an impact on you, which you had to work through, and maybe still work through because we know now, Bud, that part of your brain memorizes those things, it is part of the brain called the amygdala, where fear is stored.

And so loud voices of any kind or even loud noises can alarm you unexpectedly. Where other children who weren't exposed to that loud corporal voice would not be alarmed at other loud voices later in life, you would be. So he didn't do you any favours with his corporal voice and loud and scary voice.

So what you have to do is to digest that, and metabolize that, and you decide to forgive your dad for he didn't really have the wisdom to understand the impact that it had on his young son. So, in forgiveness, there is freedom, and you can release your anger to the wind, and just let the experience disappear into the mists of time, let it go, let go of the fear. Replace it with confidence and joy, and the idea that somehow, some way, you will handle whatever comes your way, including loud voices. Echoes from the past you'll handle your way too, and in forgiveness, you tend to erase the harshness of the experience.

Now you can go deeply into a state of comfort where you can consider ALL those remarks in your own individual way, ... so comfortable, ...so relaxed. You will be more comfortable than you've ever been for a long time with every muscle and every nerve relaxed. Now, just relax, deeper and deeper and deeper, and that's okay too. ... The deeper you relax the more comfortable you can be ... the more comfortable you are, the deeper you can relax, as deeply as you need to go, to find your answers to those experiences and come out on top. ... You can find ways of being more comfortable, emotionally and physically, with hypnosis as a way of enlisting your unconscious mind ... which is very, very powerful in its ability to make you comfortable emotionally, physically, spiritually, intellectually. Just sense yourself going d-e-e-p-e-r, d-e-e-p-e-r, and d-e-e-p-e-r so that you can you can be p-r-o-f-o-u-n-d-l-y relaxed.

In the next 15 or 20 minutes, you can review your whole life and put the story together understanding it at a deep level, so that you can feel free of fear. What a wonderful feeling that would be ... feeling free ... full of creativity, confidence, optimism ... looking forward to moments of brilliance and understanding the spiritual, physical, emotional, intellectual level ... all the episodes of your life ... You can go through your early days and easily proceed through your school years ... your adolescent years ... and pick up all the knowledge that you need how you felt in those days, and how you feel now. ... All those experiences growing up, getting bigger, wiser, older, and all the sessions you and I have had together, if you can remember all of them, it's amazing how your unconscious can track themes ... the patterns through the years becoming more and more comfortable, more and more relaxed, more creative.

You had the Tuesday nights at the hospital, you obtained the West End Police presence, [neighbourhood police] ......you worked on the cardiac pumps, you worked on projects of all kinds ... and now you are working on your book, see how it's been goal oriented ... your thoughts have been curious to explore, one of the marks of security is the ability to explore. So you made your own sense of security for yourself.

And looking at the future, Bud, if you wish to see good years coming, lots of laughter, lots of creativity, lots of feelings of epiphany when you publish this book. Lots of feelings of pride, ... lots of feelings of pleasure ... lots of feelings of your own intellectual, emotional and spiritual development in the future coming up. ... Lots of surprises that you can surprise yourself with your learning, your understanding, your compassion, your creativity ... lots of feelings of goodness from yourself to yourself. ... Intrinsically feeling well ... deep down inside ... Resting deeply and wonderfully with a refreshed restorative feeling in the morning ... And then your life can sparkle, Bud, in a way which you like ... free ... unencumbered ... hopeful ... and your feet are even comfortable when your hands are warm and soft ... Your sympathetic nervous system can take a holiday ... Your hands are warm and soft and dry ... which is a signal to your mind that your body is feeling good ... so relaxed ... so comfortable ... the deeper you go, the more comfortable you can be ... You can really be comfortable Bud, and more comfortable than you've been for a long ... long time ... what a wonderful feeling now to be that comfortable, and the comfort in that is so complete, and it's hard to understand consciously.

Stan, I phoned my sister in Winnipeg and told her about the above hypnotherapy. After I let her listen to the recording, she said emphatically, "That was mesmerizing." She actually enjoyed going into a relaxed hypnotic state. After that, we discussed the benefits of forgiving our father because he did not understand what a negative impact his loud voice had on us.

Long Term Effects of Yelling at Children

From: livstrong.com, last updated: June 18, 2015/by Lisa Mooney

Self-Confidence

It is impossible to form a healthy sense of self when you are a child who is shouted at on a frequent basis. Self-confidence depends on seeing yourself as a valued, respected and loved individual. Nemours states that kids who are shouted at can suffer damage to their self image. Children who are victims of verbal abuse rarely see themselves as worthy individuals. Their perception of themselves instead is of an insignificant being who lacks the ability to impact his society. Such children can often be helped to develop confidence by involvement in school sports or academic clubs in which they can attain self-affirmation.

Fear

Many children who are yelled at become fearful. The Women's and Children's Health Network says young children, even infants, often are frightened of loud voices particularly if these are deep, booming male voices. A timid kid might react to shouting by wincing, shaking or hiding. A long-term fearful attitude is likely to develop if the shouting abuse continues for months or years. This timidity can cause children to struggle with developing friendships. It can also impair their ability to deal with conflicts so that they withdraw from these difficult situations rather than effectively resolve them.

Concentration Problems

Concentration problems are not unusual among children who have been yelled at over a long period of time. The Children's Advocacy Center for Osceola County cites lack of concentration as one of the results of emotional abuse. Children who have learned to "tune out" shouting do so to temporarily defend themselves against the verbal assault. This defense mechanism has a negative effect later, though, as problems with focusing develop. This difficulty typically becomes an issue at school, especially in later grades where children are expected to concentrate for long periods of time. Individual attention from teachers and tutors can often help improve focus with these kids.

Taken from: W.W.W. LIVSTRONG.COM: Long Term Effects of Yelling at Children

The above knowledgeable explanation of the effect of very loud voices on children explains my experience. Hearing my father's very loud commanding voice during early childhood caused lasting generalized fear which took decades to minimize.

HORNEY, Karen (1885-1952) "Horney founded a Neo-Freudian school of psychoanalysis based on the conclusion that neuroses are the result of emotional conflicts arising from childhood experiences and later disturbances in interpersonal relationships"

From: Funk & Wagnalls New Encyclopaedia, Volume 12 page 460.

Chapter 2 - Our Family's Origin

On different dates before the First World War, my parents to be immigrated to Canada from the then Austrian-occupied area of western Ukraine. My mother arrived in Canada at age eight with her parents, two brothers, and one sister. My father came to Canada at the age of 21, along with one older brother and one younger brother, Frank. My father, Harry, had belonged to Austria's peacetime army, and managed to rise to the rank of corporal. He had a powerful, commanding, and at times threatening voice. He was a well-qualified blacksmith.

After arriving in Winnipeg, Harry decided to switch careers and so became a landscape gardener. He hired a crew of men to do landscape gardening during the summer months. The same crew also worked throughout the winter months shovelling snow from their clients' walkways, and tending to their coal-fired furnaces. Harry applied a surcharge to the hourly rate of each of his crew members. In the mid-1920s, when the accrued profit was adequate, he used the money plus a mortgage to build a two-storey grocery store at the corner of Lilac and Dudley, in the Fort Rouge area of Winnipeg. The second storey was planned for a family's living quarters. Many years later, this building was converted into apartments, and from what I have been told, it still stands today.

After approximately eight years in Canada, my father, now 29 years old, met my mother who was 14. With my maternal grandparents' consent and blessing, Harry married Carrie (Caroline). This blissful union, with its *"countless"* number of *"spring duets"*, eventually resulted in the birth of six children. Unfortunately, the first-born girl died at a very early age. The other children, in order of birth from oldest to youngest were Joe, Victoria (*"Tory"*), Ted, Vera, and David (*"Bud"*). I was born four years after Vera; therefore I had to hang around waiting for my birthday.

From what I have been told, my father spent more of his time tending to his gardening crew than serving customers in the grocery store. My mother not only served most of the store's customers, but also looked after the needs of their growing children. However, my father may have been, at times, a workaholic. Looking after his landscaping crew, soliciting new customers, and spending time in the store wasn't enough. Harry decided to add several beehives to their urban property. The neighbours nearest the bees' flight paths were not exactly ecstatic about the possibility of being stung. Fearing harm from thousands of bees, the neighbours took my father to court to sue for claimed damages caused by his notorious bees.

In court, the plaintiffs stated their case: the illegality of keeping bees within city limits, plus the claimed damages caused by my father's bees.

My father told the judge that he would agree to make total financial restitution for any damages incurred, to persons or property, provided that the plaintiffs could supply absolute proof that these damages were caused by his bees. The judge laughed, and dismissed the action as invalid for lack of evidence, in favour of the defendant. And so the bees were allowed to create honey-money for the Harry-Carrie team.

During the grocery store period, my eldest brother, Joe, ran away from home to our maternal grandparents' home. Years later, my mother told me why Joe ran away from home. Joe was told that if he did not behave, he would be forced to leave home!!!

Stan, how many children have you heard of, with a happy home life, who run away from home?

The grocery store business, from what I heard, was successful. I've been told that on occasion my father's attitude to a customer's complaint was, *"If you don't like it, shop somewhere else."* I wonder how many customers took his advice.

In the 1920s, the advent of the Safeway grocery chain introduced competition to the corner grocery stores and my parents sold their store. There may have been several reasons (of which I am unaware) for selling the grocery store, other than the Safeway competition, of course. Many corner stores were quite successful in later years.

My parents' next venture was quite a leap from a successful grocery store business to wheat farming! The 120-acre farm operation, in St. Anne, Manitoba, was, from what I was told later, a great disaster. The family stayed on their farm for approximately one year. Near the end of the farming fiasco, and with me patiently *"hanging around,"* I finally made my appearance on May 4, 1927. I sincerely believe that, under these grim farming circumstances, my arrival was as welcome as a tornado chewing the ripe wheat crop!

Later, the family farm was traded off for two houses, plus payments on the balance owing. The two houses were located approximately 26 miles from the farm, in a town called Transcona, which is now part of Greater Winnipeg. When the family moved into town on Melrose Street, I was told later, that I was a two-week-old farm boy.

Chapter 3 - A Capsule View of Our Family and Me

*S*tan, aside from the possibility of genetically inherited behaviour, I will now dwell on the psychological effects on my personality that resulted from, or have been influenced by, our dysfunctional family, relatives, and friends' interactions. I was made to feel like an insecure, homeless, penniless person, wrongly identified as the perpetrator of a criminal offence, and subsequently sentenced to a life whose full potential was corroded by fear, shame, and poverty. The result of this upbringing deepened my depressed, overly stressed, fogged, hesitant, slave-like, submissive mind, the consequences of which leaves no one, inside or outside our family, at fault or to blame!!!

The verbal abuse directed against me, as well as many traumatic psychological experiences, with threats of injury, are explained in the pages under "*Remembering.*" Some of my mind-body symptoms, resulting from these frightening traumas and verbal abuse, are:

- insomnia
- memory blocks
- painful oesophageal spasms
- overly tense muscles
- difficulty in becoming motivated
- depression
- isolation
- irritability at times

- fatigue in afternoons
- poor concentration
- difficulty in completing tasks
- shallow and stopped breath
- irritable bowel syndrome
- heart palpitations
- thoughts of death or suicide
- loss of interest in activities
- fear of social situations

My depression became an illness (clinical depression) when the symptoms described above began to interfere with the way I think and behave. Depression tends to run in families, and its cause is usually described as an imbalance of brain chemicals called neurotransmitters.

Much of our family behaviour—good, mediocre, or bad—was, I believe, learned or copied from our parents, grandparents, and significant family friends. Ours is one of many families that operated with disharmony—what we would call a dysfunctional family. What our family lacked was greater approval, nurturing, and love, and appreciation for each other. We seemed to obtain a degree of self-enhancement by degrading people, within and outside the family.

Praise was seldom given or received; fault-finding comments and insults by each insecure family member were seen as a sign of superiority, and a desirable personal necessity. Such sadistic verbal abuse gave each of us a feeling of dominance at the expense of the targeted family member by effectively lowering the self-esteem of the targeted person, while increasing the self-esteem of the abuser. These negative comments were almost invariably presented as a form of humour, combined with a contemptuous smile or arrogant grin!

The pecking order of belittling, or put-downs, came from the older family members, and were directed at the more defenceless ones, usually in birth-order sequence, with the youngest being *"the family's verbal punching bag."* Sometimes non-verbal messages were transmitted with a scowl or dirty look. And, in different ways, each family member became a victim because of our shared low self-esteem.

Some *"highlights"* from my childhood:

- *Fears* implanted in me by angry parental arguments, as early as age two.

- *Fear* instilled in me by the vicious barking dog, with teeth and saliva showing, as I tri-cycled to the grocery store and back—alone and frightened.

- *Laughed* at by both mothers (mine and the girl's), when about four years old, because one of my playmates was a girl.

- *Shamed* for over ten years by my mother and older sister because (as noted above) one of my early playmates was a girl.

- For many years, having insulting comments made to me by my two brothers and their friends, including such words such as *"booby"* (a dumb person) and *"asshole."*

- The promise of skis, which I had worked and paid for during my first job, was later broken by my mother. This broken promise was immediately followed by an insult from my sister Vera saying, *"You are too skinny to ski anyway,"* then mother and daughter turned to look at each other and broke out with broad grins! *Stan, at age sixteen, how do you think I felt?*

- Years later, the broken verbal agreement by my two brothers of the one-third profit on the sale of several real estate properties.

The above depressing remarks and broken promises left me with emotional scars. Now however, knowing these family members much better, it is difficult, but not impossible to forgive!

Chapter 4 - My Experiences as a Last Born

Stan, in order to offer you a better explanation of my behaviour and feelings, I've written about several devastating experiences in detail, some previously mentioned and not necessarily in chronological order.

For many years, I drew solely from my life experiences to explain the behaviour of others. I fell into overly simplistic *"black or white thinking,"* and fell into the trap of blaming others. I looked at how our laws and regulations are based on the premise of guilt or innocence, and how we are legally responsible for our own behaviour. I tended to use these principles to explain human behaviour, and I held rigid opinions about being *"right"* or *"wrong."* When I blamed someone for what I viewed as *"undesirable behaviour,"* I made judgment calls—despite my having no details of the person's life history, the details of which undoubtedly had a bearing on their current conduct.

The last-born child is in a unique position in the family, and it can be further affected by whether there is a variety of sexes or not because sometimes the youngest child is the parents' last chance to have a boy or a girl. In my case it probably didn't have much bearing as my parents already had two sons and two daughters.

Many cases of sibling abuse involve the youngest child being picked on, because the last born is naturally the most vulnerable. My parents and older siblings usually used me, the youngest child, to build their sense of self. My family members often belittled and ridiculed me. Of course, they knew more than I did; they were bigger and stronger; and they *"lorded over me," "the little one."* As they mocked me, my family members rewarded themselves with laughter, and thus bolstered their self-esteem. However, they also burdened me, the youngest family member, with painful, long-term memories of being shamed and humiliated by their searing verbal abuse which they brushed aside as *"just kidding."* I was born at a difficult financial time, and I wonder if I were really wanted.

The verbal abuse was essentially a kind of *"cheap way"* for my older family members, to feel powerful, important, and strong—at my expense. In our dysfunctional family, at least one source of denigration was from both my parents. My siblings copied this negative parental attitude, and so gained their parents' support and approval.

However Stan, I too must confess to exhibiting this learned, offensive, hostile behaviour (see #62 under "Remembering").

The treatment I suffered at the hands of my parents and older siblings is like the treatment meted out to young boys in fraternities when the older fraternity brothers get the younger fraternal *"initiates"* to do ridiculous things. The difference is that I was very young when family members began *"kidding"* me.

No fault.

The birth order in my family is no fault of mine, no fault of my parents and four siblings. It is just the way things were. So, as time goes on, I am slowly learning to let go of my shame, because shame is always in the eyes and judgment of other people. It all boils down to:

I am the one who knows that, in my heart, I feel worthwhile and good, and fairly compassionate. Other people's opinions of me matter less and less as I get older.

Knowing that I am a fairly decent person, the fear of being ridiculed or "*kidded*" can be overcome gradually, bit by bit. I teach my brain's amygdala that it is okay. I can do things, I can feel strong without being afraid!!! Some fear is necessary and healthy, but it should be kept in balance, adjusted depending on the situation.

The best way to overcome my fear is action, to desensitize myself bit by bit. In my case, I can overcome the fear of saying personal things in a group setting, by just saying one general thing that I can talk about, my own personal fears, and leave the specifics for a later date. So, I'll appreciate any positive feedback from people as I grow and evolve as a person. With these revelations, I am slowly leaving behind those irrational fears.

Self-comfort

I am my current age, sitting on a park bench on a lovely sunny day. Then I see myself as a seven year old walking towards me. I call out to "*young Bud*", "Come over and sit down on the bench, and we'll have a little talk." Then I say, "*Bud, even though you are frightened, humiliated, and shamed, I am here to care for you, and protect you.*" Then, I give "*little Bud*" a big hug, and feel better myself for doing so.

After talking for a while we stand up and I take *"little Bud"* by the hand. We walk to a Dairy Queen and buy two soft ice cream cones.   After several licks we become very relaxed. We walk, lick, and laugh, and feel so happy that we return to the Dairy Queen for *"seconds."*

Parental Arguments

I had the best seat in the house—my high chair, about four feet from my parents, who were seated at each end of the kitchen table—so I recall the heated arguments.

My father who immigrated from Austrian-occupied Ukraine, was formerly in the Austrian army, and had the same rank as Adolph Hitler—Corporal! My father had a very loud commanding voice, which he used frequently. When the arguments started, I must have gone into a state of shock. I didn't know why the disputes occurred, but I did know that I became petrified with fear. I was scared stiff because of the loud voices. Now my fear became well established.

When the *"discussions"* ended, my father would leave through the back door and slam it behind him in anger. Then the silence was somewhat calming and welcome. I knew there would be repeat performances, though. Fear in my future! I was always afraid of my father, a feared father figure whom I could not avoid, a terrible fear from which I could not escape, forever etched into my brain's amygdala from approximately two years of age.

Fear! Fear! Fear!

A Girl Playmate

My sister Vera had a girlfriend named Evy, (Evelyn) whose sister who was my age. These two sisters, who lived a few doors down the street, often came over to play.

Vera and Evy were of school age, and when they were at school, Nora came over to play with me. Sometimes, the girl stayed until her mother came over to fetch her for lunch.

I was about four years old at the time, and understood more English than Ukrainian, which both mothers spoke. However, when they spoke Ukrainian I did understand enough to know that they were ridiculing Nora and me. They would break out into ecstatic, almost hysterical laughter. Their painful comments and cruel laughter made me feel that having a female playmate was shameful. Laughed at when so young created long-lasting, painful memories. Nobody explained why this boy-girl playmate relationship was "*wrong*" as I interpreted it at that time.

Evy and her sister came over as playmates very often. In later years both my mother and older sister Tory, would remind me, too often, that Nora was my playmate. When either one merely mentioned the word Nora, I could see their sadistic grins as they watched for my facial expression, watched and waited for me to cringe in shame. I would turn and walk away to avoid a repetition of this painful teasing insult. I felt that having a girl playmate was improper and dishonourable. What a distorted view of reality purposely implanted in my brain!!!

Stan, the ridicule that I endured because one of my playmates was a female recurred month after month, for over a decade.

19

I felt ashamed and guilty.

My mother and sister Tory *"kidded"* me from early childhood on, for over **TEN YEARS**.

The mutual attraction of males and females—worldwide!— is a natural phenomenon, essential for the procreation of the human race!

The shaming I have described above caused me to fear taking part in this natural human experience of procreation.

So, Stan, unlike you, I am left with a hollow feeling of an unfulfilled, lost-forever family life, a lonely, childless life!

I understand now, too late, that my mother and older sister, two of the people closest to me, actually convinced me, with their tyrannical sadistic verbal abuse, that having a female playmate was *"WRONG"* and that I sincerely believed at that time in my early life period that they were "CORRECT" !!!

There were consequences as a result of this *"girl shame."*

For example, Stan, would you be surprised to learn that I had my first date with a woman when I was 23 years old!!! We only went out together once. There was nothing that I could perceive in her that was undesirable; my indelible, shameful, guilty feeling, of associating with a woman stopped the relationship.

During lunch with a group of friends, Sharon, whom I had never met before, asked me aloud to take her out. I had been told previously that Arnold, my boss sitting across from me, was Sharon's boyfriend. So I was confronted with a *"double whammy"*:

Fear of dating my boss's girlfriend.

The possibility of teasing by fellow employees.

The shame inflicted on me years earlier by my mother and sister returned to haunt me as though it were yesterday. I could not speak, I became muted, I could not say yes to a date with Sharon who had once won a Calgary beauty queen contest.

I learned later through the "*grapevine*" that because I had not dated Sharon, some people said that I must be "*gay.*"

Hell, Stan, I'm not "gay." I'm not even happy!

Sally was a secretary for a company where I was employed. It seemed obvious to me, and others, that for whatever reason, Sally was attracted to me. I took Sally out for her coffee break—only once!!! Much later, Sally moved to California and mailed a letter to me. I did not really understand why! I received a second, shorter letter from Sally, and did not reply!

Stan, employees of the company knew that I took Sally out once for coffee. I would have dated her after that only if the office staff knew nothing about it.

In my screwed-up mind, I thought that if I had taken Sally out several times, the other employees would have found out. Then I would have risked teasing, and revisiting the shame of being in a "*boy-girl*" relationship!!!

Long before I was married, I worked in the home improvement business and sometimes worked out of town. In order to reduce living expenses I decided to rent space in a residential home rather than a hotel room.

The homeowner happened to be a single female named Clara.

It turned out that Clara talked with me for a few hours. I never talked to a more pleasant woman and told her so. I was impressed by Clara and asked if we could talk again, and so we got along very well.

Later, I had to leave for Vancouver for a two month period. During this period Clara mailed a postcard to me. At this time I was living with my two elder brothers. When the postcard arrived, my brother Ted picked it up and read it. Then he handed it to me with a broad SMILE! Now, remember the opening introduction page regarding teasing, *"for some, the mere sight of a smile or hearing laughter, is enough to elicit shame, anxiety, and fear, ..."*

That did it, one SMILE by my brother had the concentrated impact equivalent to over ten years of teasing by my mother and older sister for me having one of my childhood playmates being ... A GIRL!!! It is perhaps far too difficult for most to imagine why I felt so guilty of that embedded shame, not to reply to Clara's postcard.

After two months I returned to see Clara. Now, not having communicated with Clara because of *"my guilt"*, Clara, understandably, treated me with a very cool reception – just the opposite of her initial very pleasant approach – the end of that warm relationship.

Outcast

One afternoon while I was clearing out our magazine rack, I came across a photo album made by my nephew whose mother, my sister Tory, passed away. The album included many photographs of immediate family members, close relatives, and friends.

Perhaps by now, Stan, you may not be surprised that there was an all-family photograph with one member missing, the last born, "Bud"!

Therefore, "*I am not the low man on the totem pole,*" I am not even on it, a worthless outcast! I felt total intentional rejection. Therefore I discarded the photo album into the garbage bin.

An Early Illness

While very young, I developed whooping cough (pertussis). The recurring coughing caused at least one inguinal hernia. I can faintly recall wearing a rubber-tube truss to hold the hernia bulge in place to prevent it from expanding.

I believe that having the hernia and being thin brought me more than the usual amount of attention. Being in this condition, unlike others in the family, I felt as though I was physically weaker, less than equal, not as "*good*" as the others.

The Frightened Shopper

As a preschooler with a tricycle, I was the logical "*gopher*" to send out to the local grocery store, a city block away. I felt proud of going to Polny's grocery store, the chore was family oriented and I was trusted to carry money for grocery purchases.

All went well until the Petrie family decided to acquire a medium-sized dog. This dog was allowed to run freely in their front yard behind a picket fence. The dog was not friendly. Whenever I had to shop at Polny's grocery store, and I saw that the dog was not in the yard, I tried to hurry with the purchases in the hope that the dog would still be indoors for my return trip home.

On shopping days when I passed Petrie's dog in the yard, I could see his long teeth and dripping saliva through the picket fence. The dog's barking, teeth, and saliva were very frightening for me. He appeared to be vicious.

At home, I often mentioned my fear of Petrie's dog. The reply would be a comforting, *"He won't hurt you."* Fortunately, that happened to be true for me.

Sometime later, I heard that two adult neighbours had been bitten by Petrie's dog.

Stan, imagine what that dog could have done to a small child. I was told that the police were notified of the biting dog and came to Petrie's home and put the dog down. I was relieved about the dog's demise, but my fear of it was added to my brain's amygdala.

The Cow Barn Caper

One day when I was still a preschooler, a friendly neighbour who I knew as *"Barney"*, began talking to me. He took me by the hand and led me to his family's cow barn, about a city block away.

When we arrived at the barn, it was dark inside, unlit. Barney led me to a dark corner, let go of my hand, and said in a loud, convincing voice, *"Now the cows will come in to get you"*, as he walked out of the cow barn.

With that, I burst into tears and became immobilized by fear. I stood in one spot, trembling and crying, fearing and imagining the entry of huge cows at any moment!!!

Eventually I ran out of tears and saw daylight at the barn door, left slightly ajar. I crept closely along a dark wall until I reached the door, squeezed through and walked out. Thankfully, there was not even one cow in sight!!! As I walked home alone, I thought of my close call and began to cry anew.

This frightening episode of being a lone *"captive,"* threatened by a herd of homecoming cows, became entrenched in my brain's amygdala. The amygdala is a part of the brain that retains fear and anger.

This vivid fear experience is likely one that you, can only imagine.

The Sloth

Sometimes, when company arrived, one of the topics of conversation would be my slow body movements and speech. My mother and aunt would openly compare me with one of my uncles, whose movements and speech were also slow paced. When I tried to *"correct"* myself because of this ridicule, I felt greater tension. Being the object of ridicule, by knowledgeable adults, led me to develop even lower self-esteem. I didn't feel like a *"normal human being."* I thought that something in me was *"missing."* The open mockery of my slow speech and movements taught me to limit my talking in order to avoid attracting additional derision from other people.

I believed that everything they said was the absolute truth, because I only had their opinions for reference. These people's ridicule was the opposite of what a defenceless young child requires: nourishing, accepting, and supportive treatment.

Mr. Skinner

One way my mother controlled my behaviour was with a threat. When I mentioned to her that I would like to do something that she considered improper conduct, her warning was, *"If you do, I will call Mr. Skinner and he will come over and skin you alive!!!"*

Stan, at that impressionable age I believed every word of that threat.

My behaviour was held in check by this terrorizing threat of having the skin pulled off my body—and at what cost to my psyche!!!

Years later I asked my mother if Mr. Skinner would really have *"skinned me alive."* Of course, she was *"just kidding."* Now, as an adult, I realize that without being cognizant of it, my mother unknowingly and unwittingly increased my level of fear and tension with that frightening threat.

Reading

Prior to attending school, and being the youngest of the seven family members, I was the only one who couldn't read. I was extremely determined to learn how to, and spent countless hours at the bookshelf, leafing through books, some in English and others in Ukrainian Cyrillic script.

Eventually I thought that I had *"cracked the code."* One letter, "D," in the Cyrillic script appeared to me to be a symbol. Its shape was similar to that of the living room space heater, with short legs at the bottom. I ran to my mother, asking her if I had correctly identified *"the symbol."* My mother said no, and that I would have to wait and learn how to read at school, years away in the future. Very disappointed, I returned to the bookcase with my initial depressed frame of mind. NOBODY in the family offered to teach me how to read.

It may be difficult to believe, but for decades I actually thought that I could never read a book from cover to cover!

The Student

After reading some of my experiences written so far, I think you'll understand that I acquired some unforgettable shaming over many fears.

I believe that I was *"overprotected"* by my mother because of my early illness and relatively thin body, and that may be *"normal behaviour"* for motherhood.

How many parents receive advanced training in raising children prior to having them?

I have often been accused of being *"spoiled."* Does this mean that I am responsible for my own upbringing?

Any child who is *"spoiled"* is not given adequate opportunities by their caregiver to perform basic activities. So really, the child does not learn to fend for themselves and, as a consequence, they become too dependent on their caregiver.

I remember looking forward to my first day of school—kindergarten was unavailable then. Different school teachers taught from grades 1 to 11. The school was located approximately six blocks from home.

On my first day of school, "*Bud,*" the fear-ridden six-year-old, met Miss Matheson, a kind-hearted, soft-spoken, grade one teacher. The first day of school was a sudden separation from family members that saw me left "*alone*"! I felt alone, in the presence of complete strangers, precipitating me into a feeling of extreme fear.

It may be difficult for some to believe, but I cried so often during my first year of school that I failed, the only one in our family to do so. I felt shamed and "*dumb*"!!!

Vocabulary

Many years later, my two brothers, Joe and Ted, complained to friends that when I spoke, I used words that they deemed unsuitable. Jack, a mutual friend, told me about my brothers' complaint. Jack was supportive of me, and had a discussion with Ted and Joe.

It seemed to me that anything I did or said was wrong. And perhaps, like anyone, at times I must have been "*wrong.*" However, it seemed to me that my brothers seldom—if ever—found me to be "*right*"!!! This may be another reason why, under certain circumstances, I hesitate to speak because I fear being ridiculed!

My Sibling's Compliment

Several years ago, I had abdominal surgery at UBC Hospital to have a very large intestinal polyp removed by a very skilled surgeon.

One day during my hospital convalescence, my wife Cecile, my brother Ted, his wife, Avis, and two friends, Joe and Larry, came to see me.

During their visit, a nurse came to the door to speak to me. After a short conversation, I returned to my chair. As I walked to my chair in my short hospital gown, my brother Ted said, "*Gee, you've got skinny legs!*" My visitors' silence seemed everlasting.

The Fence Walker

One fine summer day when I was a preschooler, I went into the front yard and decided to walk along the top two-by-four of the picket fence. After climbing up to the desired location, I stretched out both arms for better balance, and began a slow step-by-step walk to my destination at the end of the fence. After I had taken a few steps, my mother came out of the house in a state of panic and ordered me to climb down. Her voice really frightened me!!!

When my mother stopped me from that dangerous walk on the fence, her control of my activities didn't allow me to learn by using my own judgment about what is safe and what is dangerous. So, in a sense, this "*absolute mother control*" left me more vulnerable to danger than if I had been permitted to take part in some "*risky,*" but not too dangerous, activities. This over-control, and her doing too many things for me, extended to my being prohibited from participating in other non-threatening activities. Result? I was accused of being what some "*know-it-all people*" call "*spoiled,*" blaming the child rather than how that child's parent(s) raised them.

Reticence

While in the presence of company, my mother invariably told me to "*keep quiet.*" Perhaps this is one reason why I still have difficulty speaking to friends and acquaintances. I learned very early "*to be seen and not heard!*"

Walkman

One day my older brother Joe met me on the street while I was wearing earphones. Joe told me, "*You look terrible,*" referring to the earphones. Many people have listened to recordings in this fashion, but it was only "*I*" who looked "*terrible*" when using earphones in public.

Chapter 5 - General Attitudes to the Last Born

By a psychotherapist:

In families with children born a few years apart, it is normal that the older siblings will have grown physically stronger, become more knowledgeable, and acquired more experiences than the last-born child.

As the youngest sibling grows and matures, just as the older children did, his/her former inferior status image in physique, knowledge, and experiences is naturally going to increase. The youngest child will notice these improved mental and physical changes. Most members of the family will acknowledge these normal, slowly progressive changes in the youngest child towards adulthood. But will all family members accept and react to the youngest child accordingly? Parents and older siblings alike have to some degree a normal desire to control or influence others within realistic limits. Some may continue to see the youngest child as somewhat inferior to themselves.

The birth order of each sibling causes some degree of change in each family member's status, emotions, and parental attention. This is a normal event in family life. Of course, birth order is not the only factor to affect siblings' behaviour. Established parental interactions and attitudes, financial status, urban or rural location, and genetics also play their part.

When a newborn arrives in a family, it is normal for other siblings to feel jealous and angry. They see the newcomer being lavished with gifts and attention. Siblings require a sense of feeling, or being individual, especially with possessions, territory, clothing, etc. The youngest sibling finds it extremely difficult to share his/her property.

Along with this attention, the last born may also become the target of jokes, causing positive and negative feelings towards the same action or person, which can later result in indecision when making choices (ambivalence). *"Pecking order"* is common in mammals, humans included.

Older siblings who had complaints about their parents usually shift some of their hostility to the newborn—viewed as an invader—whom they see as siphoning off some of their former parental love, attention, and status. In an attempt to reclaim some of their former parental love and attention, certain siblings may temporarily regress to their earlier baby-like speech and behaviour.

Within legal and ethical boundaries, all children require their parents' almost unconditional acceptance and emotional support, which provides the young with a feeling of being worthy, appreciated and admired. If these emotional needs are not provided by parents, their children will gradually develop less self-confidence, low self-esteem, and more dependence. They will feel somewhat rejected and incompetent.

When nourishing acceptance and emotional support are missing, parents unknowingly or unintentionally make their children feel unworthy and insecure. The main reason for parents' lack of supportive behaviour towards their children can usually be traced back to their own childhood and upbringing. It is normal to want to be appreciated and admired by parents and siblings alike. When this does not happen, it may be sought in other possibly harmful ways.

The first six formative years of a child's life are when, it is said personality development is most strongly influenced. During these early years, children may be programmed with positive or negative perceptions of themselves, depending on the quality of family interactions and, to a lesser degree, those with significant others.

Parents who actually demonstrate reciprocal affection, cooperation, and emotional support for their spouse are more likely to receive a comparable degree of affection and support from their children. Siblings like to mimic their parents' behaviour, good or bad. Children whose emotional needs are sustained by nurturing parents develop greater self-confidence and independence, and mature into happier adults.

We expect parents to love, defend, and care for their children. Some parents who suffered painful experiences during their younger years feel that they can avoid causing similar pain in their children.

At birth, a child is naturally quite helpless. As time passes, the parent who takes an overprotective parental attitude does not allow the child to gradually learn the necessary responsibilities, as he or she ages. Why? Momma may have become the child's full-time, overindulgent, overprotective, controlling servant!!! The extreme opposite parental attitude is very little control, poor protection, and inadequate caring of their children.

In my case Stan, as previously mentioned I developed pertussis (whooping cough), at approximately two years of age, which caused a left-side inguinal hernia. I wore a truss for quite some time. I believe that because of this illness my mother overprotected me, her sickly child, for countless years.

An analogy of my overprotection is like the slave who for years was brainwashed into feeling obligated to carry out his master's orders without question. Later when freed, he is automatically geared to feel dependent on the advice of other people.

Some insecure children cannot overcome their anxiety by turning to their parents for help. Such children make unsuccessful desperate attempts to identify with a parent. Usually the mother and father struggle to master their insecurity alone, with false, inexperienced self-reliance.

So, even with this small amount of information, it can be seen that raising children to become emotionally happy, self-confident, compassionate adults, is an extremely difficult task. I asked another psychotherapist for his professional opinion on this topic. The reply:

Psychotherapist:

Extremes are damaging.

If you are overprotected, you don't have confidence in your own decision making, because you are told that you should do this and you should do that!!!

The verb "*should*" is quite damaging too, and to compare it, you can look at the other extreme: negligence versus overprotection. With negligence, those children have the problem that they feel nobody cares for them, so that neither extreme is healthy for the child.

There ought to be courses in school which focus on self-esteem, and dealing with mood and anxiety!!! I think that's just as important as math, or English, or history.

We talk about motivation—for example, how to run your life and stay focused. This depends on a fairly clearly defined set of goals. To improve your motivation, you can imagine those goals or dreams, and have them constantly before you.

Before long, they just tend to happen all by themselves because the mind works that way. It tends "*to follow its nose*," so to speak. If you direct your mind towards something specific and clear, then the energy will come!!! As Dr. Schuller used to say, "*When you have a goal and a dream it's clear that the energy just pushes forward without any effort.*" Every time you succeed, you are approaching or getting closer to your goal. You feel more energy, so that rather than wandering around and having the wind blowing you here and there, you actually don't get blown off track by the wind because you have direction!!!

Of course, the motivations that are larger than yourself are even more powerful, like you say, when you volunteered to be a senior peer counsellor. The motivation is "*pure*," in the sense that you are not being paid for it, so it's not a monetary or materialistic thing. It's just a natural inborn desire to want your life to have a larger meaning, and that really helps motivation. That's the story on motivation.

So overindulgent parents, as you say, can cause the child to be less than self-sufficient because the overindulgent parent likes to make the decisions, and, in a word, "*be bossy*" with the young child. So the child doesn't develop a sense of "*agency*" or a sense that "*he*" or "she" is making decisions, and that they are decisions that lead to consequences that are pleasing. That sense of agency, or sense of "*I am doing things,*" does not develop in the shadow of control and overindulgence. The overindulgent parent will stop kids from trying things that are at all risky, because they are afraid of the child being hurt, but when they overdo it, the paradox is that the child never learns their own judgment about what is dangerous, and what isn't, so in the end, they are more vulnerable!!!

I had a patient who grew up in a small town in Quebec, and her father wouldn't let her stay out later than 8:00 o'clock, even though she was in high school. So she eventually ran away from home when she was 18 or 19, and ended up at a bus stop in Montreal. And met a man there, who was a "*wolf*" and who saw this "*sheep*" getting off the bus, totally vulnerable. He was able to take her in easily, because she didn't know that there are dangerous people in the world, and that they can be pretty seductive: trust where trust shouldn't be given!!!

So, in the end, overindulgent parents with their fear of the child's safety cause problems with the kid's judgment of danger, and thereby decrease the child's safety as he or she grows up through the years!!!

Aside from safety issues, the child of a parent who is overindulgent becomes dependent in his or her relationships. Rather than make decisions on his/her own, he/she will ask advice of everybody. He/she won't risk making any decisions, without checking with other friends, or parents, or siblings. So he/she don't get that sense of being in control. When the people whom he/she relies on become unreliable, he/she panics!!!

On the other hand, the children who have been neglected either go one way or another. For example, they become self-sufficient. I've seen people who, at age 12, ending up parenting because the parents were very negligent. They didn't care whether their children went to school, whether they had a jacket when it was cold, whether they were well fed, or whether they were taken to the doctor when they were sick. The siblings, the smart ones, figured out that they had to take over. The downside of the children who are neglected is the fact that they feel unworthy because their parents didn't care about them.

Then they look for *"thrills"* or *"acceptance,"* or become very *"manipulative"* toward other people. Often in the extreme form they develop antisocial personality disorders, and they use substances to get a feeling that they are *"okay."*

Now, neither extreme is good for the child. The middle-of-the-road policy is always the best where the parent will take some risks with the child in order for the child to feel that that he/she has a sense of who he/she is, and a sense of agency (of being in action or exerting influence).

The parent allows the child to make mistakes and is not too judgmental. They allow the child to broach some dangerous things, and then perhaps, rescue them, if they are getting into real trouble. They'll let them get into a bit of trouble, knowing that's the only way they really learn to avoid trouble, by actually avoiding *"some trouble."*

Children have to experience some pain in order to discover it.

Parents who are *"in the middle of the road"* realize that kids have to find out that life is good, but sometimes it is not so good. That's the most realistic appraisal that helps children go through the world, without getting too disappointed when things don't go well or, on the other hand, too Pollyanna, or optimistic, when things go well. So, the middle of the road is what they are hoping for.

As we talked about last time, Bud, the fact that we don't learn things in school like parenting, and the vulnerabilities of the youngest born, or notions of sibling abuse, is really inexcusable, since parenting is such a fundamental responsibility and privilege!!!

Stan, A Few Last-Born Characteristics:

- Creative.
- Sensitive.

- Immature.
- Caring.
- Secretive.
- Can exhibit erratic behaviour.
- Can become too eager.
- Affectionate.
- Idealists.

Some Famous Last-Born People:

- Bill Gates.
- Howard Stern.
- Jay Leno.
- RalphNader

Chapter 6 - Effects of Family Interactions on Children

*S*tan, the following is what I learned from one of my psychotherapists: I am now aware that the formative six years of my life strongly influenced the development of my personality.

Parents, older siblings, and family friends can, without realizing it, transfer some of their patterns of perception and behaviour and their own conditioning to young children. So, during these early years, depending on the quality of family interactions, children may be programmed with positive or negative perceptions of themselves. Because young children like to imitate or copy adult actions, speech, etc. (often as play or teasing), this early learning becomes part of their developing behaviour patterns.

When parents can actually demonstrate their reciprocal affection, mutual cooperation, and emotional support, each spouse has feelings of worth, appreciation, and love. Also, having (or striving for) such healthy and harmonious relationships tends to dampen the severity of future differences of opinion that are bound to arise.

Children raised by such parents are more likely to receive greater affection and support. These children, in turn, will likely mimic some of their parents' behaviour.

When these emotional needs are sustained by nurturing parents, their children feel worthy, admired, and loved. Such children gradually develop greater self-confidence and independence, and, in time, ripen into happier adults.

All children require both parental and sibling acceptance, including emotional support, feeling worthy, and feeling loved. When these emotional needs are not satisfied, they may be sought within or outside the family, sometimes in ways that are unhealthy or harmful to the self or to others. The process of raising children is affected by parents' personalities, relative experience or inexperience, financial status, etc. The job of successfully raising a family can be very difficult.

When domineering parents use ridicule, criticism, and faultfinding on their children, they can unknowingly or unwittingly make their children feel unworthy, unloved, lonely, and depressed. The reason for parents' lack of supportive behaviour towards their children can usually be traced back to their own childhood upbringing.

The biggest favour parents can do for their children is to be loving to each other—it is unspoken, but it is there—that is, love in the home!!!

Ideally, parents can show affection or love for their children by being:

- Encouraging
- Gentle
- Forgiving
- Non-judgmental
- Patient
- Humorous
- Adventurous

And:

- Having faith in their children
- Supporting their children in trusting their own intuition
- Suppressing sibling-to-sibling abuse
- Participating in their children's lives, e.g., attending soccer games
- Modelling parental marital bliss
- Avoiding parental threats, ridicule, and verbal and physical abuse

Unfortunately, not all parents demonstrate this *"love in the home"* pattern, often because they did not receive much of it in their own childhood years.

Now, Stan, in this true life example, you can come to your own conclusion as to how my former schoolmate was raised.

While in grade 7, John K. frequently came to the classroom with red eyelids. Sometimes John entered the room crying, and told us how his parents treated him.

One day John K. asked Sam S. and me to meet him at Tony's Café after school for coffee. During our conversation, John reached into his pocket and pulled out a pistol, not a toy. Sam and I wondered why John had brought the gun. Later, we learned that John had become a hit man for Winnipeg's underworld.

Many years later, John moved to Vancouver. I don't know how it was arranged, but John was incarcerated without a criminal charge!

Guess what, Stan? John was sent to the maximum security wing of Oakalla Prison Farm where I was employed at the time. John was extremely angry about being put in jail without being charged with an offence. Under these circumstances I avoided any contact with him.

Later, after his release from jail, John went to a Hastings Street beer parlour where he was shot to death by an assassin who was sitting at his table!!!

Stan, I asked another psychotherapist to give his opinions on proper parenting:

Psychotherapist:

It's known now that being parented properly gives you a head start in life. Touching, holding—loving is such a fundamental experience required for feeling secure. Why is that topic not addressed in schools to young kids who will eventually become parents? Some of them who are taught what good parenting is all about may even reflect that they can teach their parents one thing or two things about their side of being parented.

It could be an interesting dynamic about what it's like for them to parent while the kids are thinking, now how is it going to be for me to parent, given my experience of being parented. So the principles are not difficult to understand: when a child is secure, the child explores. When the child is insecure, the child doesn't explore the world. So a sense of security is fundamental to a child exploring the world which, as a child grows up into an adult, is a trait that sticks with them through the years. So that fear is experienced in proportion to real danger, not danger from a false sense of insecurity.

Other things that the parents can teach children by osmosis, you might say, is that when the parents have a good relationship between themselves, it sinks into the kids about what a good relationship is all about.

So, kids in school who will be parents some day, can learn that when they marry, they should try their level best to pick somebody who is steady and true, because it's fundamental to raising children to give you an example of a secure, trustworthy relationship.

Another thing the parents can give their kids is a sense of joy. Joy in an ordinary thing, everyday things, so that instead of being fearful or obsessive or anxious or depressed, they move through life with a sense of joy, a sense of ever-blissfulness.

A sense of meaning to give kids the message that they need to create their own meaning in life is another principle. Something worthy outside themselves is usually the approach that we all need. The parents in their teaching can help their children get a sense of accomplishment—achieve something, ... that they can actually operate in the world and find that they get results.

Another trait that can be explored with children is the sense of creativity, thinking "out of the box," and even simple things can teach kids that sort of thing.

Humour is creative, to tell a joke is a creative experience, for example.

To tell the kids about the German chemist F.A. Kekule, who discovered the benzene ring ... Finally, whole numbers of doors were opened in chemistry when Kekule realized that carbon compounds don't have to exist in a straight line, they can actually exist as a ring.

As a parent, you can actually teach kids how to be creative. You ask them what use can be made of an umbrella other than keeping rain off you. Well, then kids will say, "*It can keep sun off you too*," and that is true. Then you can turn it upside down and carry a few items in it if you didn't have a bag—and onward in terms of making kids appreciate creative thinking.

These are not difficult concepts, and you can weave them into kids' lives by asking them, "*Can you give me an example of what it feels like to be at home where there is a lot of warmth and laughter and not much judgement or criticism?*" So they have an insight into how they would like to be parented and they can actually do that when they actually become parents.

These are just some of the principles that could be introduced with some colour commentary along the way and make the kids laugh as they learn, because people learn better when they are relaxed and laughing.

The kids can do their own projects: What do you do with a kid who is rebellious? What do you do with a kid who procrastinates? So, you can set up a bunch of problems and let the kids find ways of solving problems that typically parents deal with. You can have a workshop on that subject and the kids can bring up examples knowing that they sometimes get rebellious and sometimes procrastinate.

It can be a dynamic learning class, probably 8, 9, 10 years of age is a good time to start, and maybe dip into it every year for a few hours here and there.

When the children get into the grade 11 to 12 period, they can tackle more complex issues such as boundaries between parents and children such as people who are oppressive, or people who are too permissive or blaming and so forth.

The early years can fold into the later years as school goes on with more complex subjects, as I don't think it would steal much time from math, physics and chemistry. I think it could help the kids learning and then help their kids, so it is a very future-oriented kind of thinking going on here.

Chapter 7 - On Parenting

Compare the following information on parenting with my upbringing, where fear was instilled in me to control my behaviour. For example: *"If you do not behave, Mr. Skinner will come over and skin you alive!"* The threats of bodily harm used by my mother worked, but she wasn't aware of the toll it exerted on my psyche. Another psychotherapist on parenting:

Psychotherapist:

We are talking about parenting and some of the principles of good parenting, and how to teach children before they get too biased on these principles.

These are some thoughts, Bud, about parenting and teaching kids to parent. These are some thoughts generated from the book NurtureShock by Po Bronson and Ashley Merryman.

How to make it stick by role playing certain scenarios. How to envision children ages 10, 11, 12, perhaps each year having a theme. First year would be to teach kids how to have a loving family structure, where the children are respected, and there is honesty about feelings, and you can be angry, but then you look how to work things through without getting too angry.

In other words the process of solving problems and you could role play that.

Then the next year could focus on ethics which includes honesty, and knowing right from wrong.

Perhaps the next year, more subtle things that the kids could pick up in their more mature years, such as parents not being too permissive, and that delicate way of walking the middle of the road where kids aren't confused in the sense that they don't have to rebel against too much strictness, nor do they have to rebel against not enough guidelines.

Then the next year, the whole idea of the structure of a good family could be discussed by how parents reflect in their own relationships, how to get along, and the idea that the best favour you can give to your children is a good relationship between Mom and Dad, because it percolates down all the way through. So, if the children notice the parents treating each other with respect, enjoying good humour, love, affection, being creative, being the kind of people who are admired by their peers and friends ...

Perhaps the next year, you could look at the families and have a sense of community at large. Many parents are too insular, then kids become insular and not connected. So you want to have a family that is integrated with the community.

So, all these principles could be taught through the years. Some of the more subtle principles could be taught in the later years, when the children are able to understand walking a fine line between permissiveness and strictness. This is a concept that really requires some maturity and advanced thinking.

Perhaps even in high school, children could be taught about:

- What is a nuclear family, and how does it relate to the family of origin?

- How does it communicate to the community at large, and what is the history of the nuclear family?

- What is happening to the family in our society, with 50% divorce rate?

- Blended families, the whole notion even though you know the parents are split, and the other one is remarried, that somehow or other they remain friends. They are able to understand how to integrate and blend with their respective families. Also keep some sense of civility, friendliness, and caring between the blended members of each family.

So here is a bit of addition, where one principle would be, as I mentioned previously, that the concepts need to be age sensitive. Starting at the top, I think grade twelves would be sufficiently equipped to understand how a family would be part of a community. That is to say, the children would have encouragement "*to stretch their wings*" and belong to various groups. The parents would help their children to understand the nature of healthy relationships.

Obviously when the children are exposed too much about the world, or exposed to good and bad, safety is a cardinal thing. An example of that, in the sense of giving the kids a good example, is that parents have always told the kids, be careful what you put in your mouth, be careful what you eat. So the message is, when it comes to things like drugs which are substances that you don't exactly know what they are, simply abstain. Therefore, kids in the home where they've always been taught to be careful what you put in your mouth would not likely get involved with drugs.

Also, if the parents never get drunk, that would be another way of giving their children a message to be careful about alcohol. So that would be a theme for grade 11 and 12 children to understand.

Further safety issues are things like driving. Good parents would teach their kids, or have their kids attend safe driving schools. One of the major dangers children face, apart from drugs, is driving.

Another concern of parents should be their children's emotional life. In other words, if they identify with anxiety and depression, they should watch for signs of it in their children. Each of the children should be given the chance to talk to their parents. So a trusting relationship could develop where the children feel comfortable talking to parents about their problems. Parents can help their children solve issues—often it is relationship issues.

One of the most devastating things that kids may have to deal with, besides drugs and driving is the break-up of relationships. Parents should talk to their children about how relationships begin, how the middle part goes, and sometimes how it ends. Also, how then to cope with such an ending?

Another area, of course, is discipline. Such training is learned by the way children handle their studies, eating, and exercise. The best way to teach children those things would be in a non-verbal way about studying properly, eating right, and exercising right. Parents can impart these very important messages to their children.

Further areas are pacing, and one of your favourites, Bud, is not rushing. So, you teach your kids not to rush, to take time to enjoy the tasks, and take breaks, and have a good sense of rhythm.

Sleep and rest are other things that you teach your children to respect their body rhythm, so that they take adequate rest along with adequate exercise.

Then some of the more subtle areas of creativity, as you say, when the children come up with notions that they want to do something, like in your case, Bud, read when you were young. That's a good opportunity for the parents to appreciate the child's creativity, and nurture it right from the start.

So, age-related lessons should be focused on the younger children, who need help in developing a sense of confidence in themselves. Parents are often quick to praise but should also give their children adequate and real feedback when they don't do things the right way. Parents should spend time on children's interaction with their school activities. They should spend time meeting the teacher and figuring out how to fine-tune the children's adjustment at school, whether or not they are applying themselves.

Often the good teachers tell parents how their children are getting along with other children. I call it "*the fine-tuning concept*," where kids are overly friendly because they desire positive reinforcement. Also when they are less friendly and are a bit shy, the parents help the teacher help the child. At home, parents, of course, talk to the child about reaching out and enjoying other people.

You can identify areas of accomplishment, and how children can set goals and how important it is to have goals. The dangerous time in one's emotional life is when you've not set goals, or you are between goals. Setting goals is almost like walking down a path: if you know where you are going, the wind, even though it blows, doesn't blow you off the path. If you are not sure where you are going, then it blows you off the path.

So, talking to children about their general life goals, what they dream about, what they are passionate about, is an amazing thing to do as a parent. You realize through the years that the children are able to absorb principles. Children also need to be taught ethics, what is right or wrong and how to do the right thing in the right way.

A good example is where there are no lies, agendas, or secrets among the family members. So the children grow up in a trusting environment, and in that way they learn to trust.

You have to be very careful to nurture trust with yourself and with others. Of course, loving is the bottom line of it all, and loving means you are happy that other people are happy.

So, you teach your children to reach out and be glad when other people are doing well.

Parents must teach their children not to compare themselves with other children because each person is unique, and has his or her own way of being in the world. It feels special and unique and is a wonderful thing to teach children.

Another psychotherapist reviewed *NurtureShock*, by Po Bronson and Ashley Merriman.

Po Bronson, MFA, BA, has published six books; written for TV, magazines, newspapers (including the *New York Times*, Wall Street Journal, and National Public Radio's Morning Edition); made a social documentary bestseller called What Should I Do With My Life; and his novel *Bombardiers* was a number one bestseller in the United Kingdom. His books have been translated into nineteen languages!

Authors Po Bronson and Ashley Merriman, BA, have received:

- The American Association for the Advancement of Science for best journalism.

- The Mensa Award.
- The Clarion Award for the best magazine feature.
- The Council on Contemporary Families for Outstanding Journalism.

Both authors are currently writing *NurtureShock* columns for Nesweek.com

Chapter 1

The chapter talks about the inverse power of praise, where parents say children are really "*good.*" They are faced with the test, and they bow out, because they don't want to be "*good.*" Whereas the other parents said you are "*good*" and you have to work hard to do things. The work ethic is important, and those children did well in tests. So it is an interesting concept that the simple repeated praise can actually inhibit children's self-esteem.

Chapter 2

The next chapter was about sleep and how important it is to get adequate sleep. If you don't get enough sleep, you might suffer the consequences of decreased IQ, less emotional well-being, and perhaps ADHD and obesity. There have been a lot of studies over the years about the results of children who are sleeping six to seven hours, versus the ones sleeping eight to nine hours. The latter group do much better on all tests. So it appears that the human brain needs that rest period to perform well.

This sleep hygiene which is taught later in life can be taught earlier in life. The children could benefit from it and realize that when they eventually have children they could teach them sleep hygiene. Essentially sleep hygiene is turning down the activity level in your mind and your behaviour. Therefore, don't exercise in the evening and don't look at newscasts later in the evening. Develop a ritual of going to sleep with learned relaxation techniques and this might result in a wonderful rejuvenating kind of sleep.

Chapter 3

Chapter 3 is about race. It is a fascinating chapter because the authors talk about not talking to the children about race but then, of course, it comes up anyway. The conclusion is that it is better to talk openly with children about race, and sex, and so forth. So when the children are talked to in that way by teachers, they will now experience openness about race, sex, and so forth, and parents can teach their children that too.

Chapter 4

Chapter 4 is about children who lie. It's so interesting that when children are being videotaped and they are lying about something, it is difficult to determine the truth. Even policemen do no better than chance in terms of telling whether children lie or not. It's interesting that the more socially skilled children are better liars. It's kind of an interesting thought that children are skilled at lying as well.

Chapter 5

In search of intelligent life in kindergarten children is the next chapter. This sentence in this chapter is fascinating. "*If you picked a hundred kindergarten children as gifted, i.e., the smartest, by third grade, only 27 of them would still deserve that categorization.*" You would have wrongly locked out 73 other deserving students. So the tests are poor predictors. I think the moral of this chapter is that their tests should be given through the years. They may or may not predict their outcomes in terms of excellence. So that when children become parents, they can put testing in a good context for their children.

Chapter 6

The next chapter is the sibling effect. In this chapter it says that Freud was wrong and Shakespeare was right. That means that Freud's theory that a lot of fighting with siblings was trying to get parental attention and love. But this seems to be last on the list of priorities for children. First on the list of priorities is who's got what toy, who's got what privilege to play in the living room, in terms of the best chair, and these kinds of things are important. It seems true that if you are the youngest child, you are going to get abuse no matter what happens. It is safer to give you, the younger child, abuse because the likelihood is that there is no retribution.

So now children can talk to their children, when they become parents, about sharing. And I know that looking at groups like the Beavers, for example, the major theme that the Beavers have is sharing. So the whole concept of sharing in preschools is important.

Children are taught by preschool teachers to share the little bicycle, or share the blocks and so forth. So these are very important lessons to learn.

Now, in modern society, much of business activities, for example, is conducted by teams. So to be a team player is a very interesting and critical thing to learn as children. Children could learn that, and when they learn that, they learn that they can teach their children in turn.

Chapter 7

Chapter 7 is called *"The Science of Teen Rebellion."* It is an interesting concept that teenagers need to rebel in our society. Their rebellion is part of them, defining themselves vis-à-vis their parents and their parents' values.

In terms of being a parent, it is good to be flexible, although there must be boundaries for your children. It's a delicate fine line between being rigid and too permissive. It's a judgemental call continuously, and there are no easy answers to it. But as parents, we want to foster our children's sense of themselves, and so we have to tolerate some rebellion. Rebellion might include, for example, living a more relaxed lifestyle. Some of the parents are, in the view of the teenagers, working too much and their balance between work and pleasure is askew.

Certainly, some of the younger students coming out of university have redefined the balance between work and non-work life.

Another issue that teenagers rebel about is restriction in terms of freedom to pursue things like drugs, gambling, and sex. Of course, the parents have to provide firm boundaries and values for their teens in those areas.

Young people need to have something to bounce off. We don't want children defining themselves as the negative of their parents.

Hopefully you can allow children to contemplate different kinds of lifestyles, not just the opposite of the parents.

Rebellion is a positive thing. In other cultures rebellion is discouraged. Values are to be obedient to their culture. Human civilization has evolved beyond those parameters.

Chapter 8

Chapter 8 is very interesting. It writes about the concept called Tools, or more properly, Tools of the Mind. This is a way of teaching which includes role playing, and kids taking individual parts in a play, such as Fire Station. They measured the results of the programs and the children came out way ahead, which to me, is an example of parenting with imagination, storytelling.

Deepak Chopra talked about telling their children cliff-hanging stories and asking them to complete the stories in the morning.

Dr. Sylvia Bunge, neuroscientist at the University of California, Berkeley, looked at the brain in the rostral lateral prefrontal cortex region, responsible for maintaining concentration and setting goals. Tools of the Mind seems to wire up the right lateral prefrontal cortex which is a neuroscience confirmation that Tools of the Mind have a major impact. These approaches would be something that parents learn with their children.

Chapter 9

Chapter 9, *"Why Modern Involved Parenting Has Failed to Produce a Generation of Angels."* There were astonishing results with Ostrov's team when they found out that educational programs increased the aggressive behaviour in children. They discovered that educational programs first of all had to set up a conflict in terms of relationship, and then solve it. In setting the stage they were modelling overly assertive behaviour, another kind of counterintuitive scientific discovery.

Another counterintuitive scientific finding was that progressive dads weren't as good as traditional dads in counselling their children. The progressive dads were probably a little too involved in their children's lives and had poor marital relationships in general. It is very interesting when science digs down on concepts.

Chapter 10

This chapter talks about the need for children to have live parents rather than videos teaching them language. There is no substitute for human interaction. We could teach children in school about parenting and how vital it is to have human interaction versus electronic interaction.

Conclusion

The concluding chapter, amid the myth of the super traits or gratitude. They talk about new approaches strengthening positive emotions such as resilience, happiness, and gratitude. They talk about students keeping a gratitude journal, and they were 25% happier than when they didn't keep the journal.

It appears that gratitude is a very highly evolved emotion. When one thinks about gratitude, it generates many positive corollary aspects to human nature.

Children need to understand that they have a gift when their parents provide them with a good environment, and teachers make sacrifices for the good of the children. Gratitude intervention works, even with the youngest children.

Teaching children parenting has a great advantage. It breaks the cycle of emotional, physical, or even sexual abuse from going down the generations, as it could do, if children don't learn proper parenting skills at an early age.

That's it, Bud.

Nine Steps to More Effective Parenting

Stan, we are often told from many sources how to raise our children, the following steps contain very sound advice.

1. Boosting Your Child's Self-esteem.

- Your words and actions as a parent affect their developing self-esteem more than anything else.

- Praising accomplishments, however small, will make them feel proud. By contrast, belittling comments or comparing a child unfavourably with another will make kids feel worthless.

- Comments like "What a stupid thing to do!" or "You act more like a baby than your little brother!" cause damage just as physical blows do.

- Let your kids know that everyone makes mistakes and that you still love them, even when you don't love their behaviour.

2. Catch Kids Being Good

- You may find yourself criticizing far more often than complimenting.

- The more effective approach is to catch kids doing something right.

- *"I was watching you play with your sister and you were very patient!"* These statements will do more to encourage good behaviour over the long run than repeated scoldings.

- Be generous with your rewards - your love, hugs, and compliments can work wonders.

3. Set Limits and Be Consistent With Your Discipline

- The goal of discipline is to help kids choose acceptable behaviours and learn self-control.

- They may test the limits you establish for them, but they need those limits to grow into responsible adults.

- Your house rules helps kids understand your expectations and develop self-control. e.g. no TV until homework is done, no hitting, no name-calling or hurtful teasing allowed.

- You can't discipline kids for talking back one day and ignoring it the next. Being consistent teaches what you expect.

4. Make Time for Your Kids

- It is often difficult for parents and kids to get together for a family meal, and there is probably nothing kids would like more.

- Kids who aren't getting such attention they want from their parents often act out or misbehave because they're sure to be noticed that way.

- Create a 'Special Night' each week to be together, and let your kids help decide how to spend the time.

- Attending concerts, games, and other events with your teen communicates caring and lets you get to know your child and his or her friends.

- Don't feel guilty if you're a working parent. Little things you can do – making popcorn, playing cards, window shopping – that kids love.

- Talk to your child every day about what went well and what was difficult.

5. Be a Good Role Model

- Young kids learn a lot about how to act by watching their parents.

- Be aware that you're being watched by your kids. Studies have shown that children who hit, usually have a role model for aggression at home!

- Above all, treat your kids the way you expect other people to treat you!!!

6. Make Communication a Priority

- You can't expect kids to do everything simply because you, as a parent, *"say so."* They want and deserve explanations as much as adults do.

- Make your expectations clear. If there is a problem invite your child to work on solutions and consequences with you.

- Make suggestions. Kids who participate in decisions are more motivated to carry them out.

7. Be Flexible and Willing to Adjust Your Parenting Style

- If you often feel "let down" by your child's behaviour, perhaps you have unrealistic expectations.

- Parents who think in "should" might find it helpful to read up on the matter or to talk to other parents or child development specialists.

- As your child changes, you'll gradually have to change your parenting style. Chances are, what works with your child now, won't work as well in a year or two.

8. Show That Your Love Is Unconditional

- When you have to confront your child, avoid blaming, criticizing, or fault-finding, which undermine self-esteem and can lead to resentment.

- Make sure they know that although you want and expect better next time, your love is there no matter what.

9. Know Your Own Needs and Limitations as a Parent

- You have strengths and weaknesses as a family leader.

- Try to have realistic expectations for yourself, your spouse, and your kids. You don't have to have all the answers – be forgiving of yourself.

- Focus on the areas that need the most attention rather than trying to address everything all at once.

- Take time out from parenting to do things that will make you happy as a person (or as a couple).

- Focusing on your needs does not make you selfish. It simply means you care about your well-being, which is another important value to model for your children.

From: *http://kidshealth.org/parent/positive/family/nine_steps.html*

Ten Reasons Not to Hit Your Kids

by Jan Hunt

In 37 countries around the world* it is illegal for a parent, teacher, or anyone else to spank a child, and 113 countries prohibit corporal punishment in schools.

The most important reason for banning physical punishment of children, according to Dr. Peter Newell, coordinator of the organization End Punishment of Children, is that *"all people have the right to protection of their physical integrity, and children are people too."*

1. Hitting children teaches them to become hitters themselves.

2. In many cases of so called *"bad behaviour"*, the child is simply responding in the only way he can, given his age and experience. For this reason, punishment is not only ineffective in the long run, it is clearly unjust.

3. Punishment distracts the child from learning how to resolve conflict in an effective and humane way. A punished child becomes preoccupied with feelings of anger and fantasies of revenge, and is thus deprived of the opportunity to learn effective methods of solving the problem at hand. Thus, a punished child learns little about how to handle or prevent similar situations in the future.

4. Punishment interferes with the bond between parent and child, as it is not human nature to feel loving toward someone who hurt us. In contrast, cooperation based on respect will last permanently, bringing many years of mutual happiness as the child and parent grow older.

5. Many parents never learned in their own childhood that there are positive ways of relating to children. When punishment does not accomplish the desired goals, and if the parent is unaware of alternative methods, punishment can escalate to more frequent and dangerous actions against the child.

6. Punishment may appear to produce "*good behaviour*" in the early years, but always at a high price, paid by parents and by society as a whole, as the child enters adolescence and early adulthood.

7. Spanking on the buttocks, an erogenous zone in childhood, can create in the child's mind an association between pain and sexual pleasure, and lead to difficulties in adulthood.

8. Blows to the lower end of the spinal column send shock waves along the length of the spine, and may injure the child. Lower back pain among adults in our society may well have its origins in childhood punishment. Some children have become paralyzed through nerve damage from spanking.

9. Physical punishment gives the dangerous message that *"might makes right"*, that it is permissible to hurt someone else, provided they are smaller and less powerful than you are. The child then concludes that it is permissible to mistreat younger or smaller children.

10. Because children learn through parental modeling, physical punishment gives the message that hitting is an appropriate way to express feelings and solve problems.

"Gentle instruction", supported by a strong foundation of *"love and respect"*, is the only truly effective way to bring about commendable behaviour, instead of *"good behaviour"* based only on *"fear."*

Sweden, Finland, Norway, Austria, Cyprus, Denmark, Latvia, Croatia, Bulgaria, Israel, Germany, Turkmenistan, Iceland, Ukraine, Romania, Hungary, Greece, Netherlands, New Zealand, Portugal, Uruguay, Venezuela, Spain, Togo, Costa Rica, Republic of Moldova, Luxemburg, Lichtenstein, Poland, Tunisia, Kenya, Republic of Congo, Albania, South Sudan, Macedonia, Honduras, and Malta. (Source: Global Initiative to End Corporal Punishment of Children)

From: www.naturalchild.org/tenreasons.html

Stan, when do you think that teaching people proper parenting would result in greater success for their children:

(a) before they became parents?

(b) or after they became parents?

Chapter 8 - Hypnosis

The information below is taken from conversations with two psychotherapists.

History

The technique of hypnosis has been used in somewhat different forms and by many world religions for many centuries. Around the mid-19th century hypnosis was used in India as an anesthetic during surgery. This came to an end with the advent of chloroform and ether.

Dr. F.A. Mesmer, born in 18th-century Austria, is said to be the *"father of hypnosis."* Dr. Mesmer referred to his hypnosis as *"animal magnetism."* He actually used magnets to supposedly realign fluids in the human body in order to cure illnesses. At that time, hypnosis was known as mesmerism.

Dr. James Baird, a Scottish physician who has also been called the *"father of hypnosis,"* was the first to use the term *"hypnosis."* He believed that the state of being in a trance was a form of sleep, and so he named the phenomenon after Hypnos (Greek god of sleep). Baird claimed that magnets were not necessary to produce an altered state of mind—that is, a hypnotic trance.

In 1893 the British Medical Association claimed that the state of hypnosis could have beneficial effects for humans. And Dr. Sigmund Freud used hypnosis around the same time until he developed his psychoanalytic procedures.

In the 20th century, the American Dr. Milton Erickson became the leading proponent of hypnotherapy. Dr. Erickson treated his patients by getting them to focus into their subconscious minds, and he also noted their non-verbal communications.

Hypnosis and Hypnotherapy

Hypnosis and hypnotherapy work when a person accepts suggestions from either the hypnotist or *"the self."* All hypnosis is essentially self-hypnosis. It is a natural way to improve our behaviour and health, and to bring us into a more relaxed frame of mind.

Hypnosis is defined as an altered state of consciousness (unlike sleep), characterized by a heightened susceptibility to suggestion. The hypnotist gets the attention of the subject and suggests certain tasks in a slow, calm voice.

The instructions generally include muscle relaxation, breathing, and other needs of the subject. As the subject goes into a trance-like state, he/she absorbs himself/herself with his/her inner thoughts and feelings. The subject reflects on what he/she sees during this experience. Most people can be hypnotized, but the depth of the trance will range from a light to deep hypnotic state. Even a light trance offers valuable therapeutic effects.

During hypnosis there is:

- an easing of stress or tension, with feelings of relaxation;
- a heightened suggestibility to instructions; and
- a deeper contact with the subject's emotional life and buried fears.

Tension has a negative physical and psychological effect on individuals, and inhibits the body's healing responses. Stress reduction through hypnosis can benefit certain cases of:

- High blood pressure
- Coronary heart disease
- Asthma
- Migraine headaches
- Digestive disorders
- Menstrual difficulties
- Skin ailments

Hypnotic suggestions can assist in the elimination of:

- A smoking habit
- Insomnia
- Overeating
- Amnesia
- Paralysis
- Fugue state (a disturbed, seemingly conscious state which includes amnesia)
- Visual, hearing, and speech disorders
- Enuresis (involuntary passing of urine)
- Impotence
- Malnutrition

Some common hypnotic experiences that are examples of hypnotic-like states:

- When a football player suffers an injury during a game, he may continue to play without realizing that his injury occurred.
- When time seems to *fly by* and you don't know why.

- When you travel a very commonly used route, you may have little recall of the scenery or the actual trip—this indicates how common hypnosis really is, and most of us experience it without realizing.

In a conscious state of mind, a person may believe that he/she is not totally aware; that is, not really on the ball or not as sharp as possible, sluggish. Hypnosis (an altered state of consciousness) allows a person to reach the subconscious mind. And while in a subconscious state, a person's former belief barriers can be transformed into new and improved thinking and behaviour patterns. It really is a very powerful and useful process.

Hypnotherapy is believed to work when a person enters a trance state of mind, the analytical side of the brain relaxes, and the creative side of the brain then takes over. Another theory is that it is a matter of the patient being willing to accept suggestions, and desiring to heal his/her illness.

A key principle is that our minds work at different conscious levels, and during hypnosis the conscious mind is put on standby, allowing the subconscious mind to become highly susceptible to suggestions from the hypnotist. Practitioners say that it is not possible to hypnotize someone against his/her will because the subconscious mind is forceful and will not accept unreasonable suggestions. Similarly, if the patient is uncomfortable with the psychotherapist, the patient may resist the psychotherapist's instructions.

Stan, during hypnotherapy, the psychotherapist would ask you in a slow, soothing, relaxed voice to sit or lie down, relax, and close your eyes. The psychotherapist would then ask you to relax *your muscles and to visualize yourself relaxing on a beautiful beach, the sun's rays warming your body, with pleasant music in the background. You are totally conscious during this therapy.*

The psychotherapist's purpose is to help your mind enter a deeper relaxed state, or trance, in which your mind begins to heal itself, with the psychotherapist's suggestions, of whatever your body is afflicted with.

As previously mentioned, the trance state improves your imagery and your ability to focus your attention on the psychotherapist's suggestions, which can help to improve on such psychosomatic conditions as:

- Food/alcohol/drug addictions
- Depression
- Fears and shame
- Insomnia
- Stress
- Skin conditions

Hypno-sedation

Dr. Marie Elisabeth Faymonville, of Belgium, now world renowned, pioneered the use of hypno-sedation to replace general anesthetics. Faymonville, together with her team of doctors, have to date performed over 5,000 surgeries under hypno-sedation.

Hypno-sedation is the combined use of hypnosis and sedative/local anesthetic in surgery instead of general anesthetic. Patients undergoing hypno-sedation experience much fewer side effects than patients given general anesthetics and are able to return to work in approximately half the time of patients who had a general anesthetic. Unfortunately, not all patients can be put into a hypnotic trance.

Hypnosis is used for pain control in childbirth, dentistry, and surgery. However, hypnosis cannot match the reduction of pain offered by chemical anesthetics. What it can do is raise the pain threshold to a point where only a small fraction of the chemical anesthetic is necessary to obtain the equivalent reduction of pain.

My Hypnosis Experiences

Stan, read all three hypnotic trances slowly and calmly.

Example One: Entering the first hypnotic trance for my foot pain:

Psychotherapist:

The basic principle of hypnosis is learning to relate to your unconscious mind. Dr. Erickson used to say, "*your unconscious mind knows much more than you do.*" One of the interesting things you can do with self-hypnosis is pain control. You can even use the concept of post-hypnotic suggestion. That is to say, in your trance you can say, "*Can my unconscious mind find a way for me to be comfortable even after I awaken?*" In your case, Bud, you might think of putting your aching feet in a trance along with the rest of you. Upon waking up, leave your feet in a trance. So that is a kind of post-hypnotic suggestion: even though you are awake, your feet remain in a trance.

You can be comfortable while the doctors are exploring the exact cause, whether it is peripheral neuropathy, or irritation of the nerves, or whether it is muscle pain, or it is joint pain associated with arthritic pain, or some combination of those things.

You might want to check your sugar, and check with your rheumatologist, to rule out some of those possibilities. But in the meantime, using your talents of hypnosis you can be exquisitely sensitive to your unconscious mind which knows what to do because for most of your life, you haven't been aware of your feet. They were just there, and wouldn't that be wonderful not to be aware of your feet, and be more aware of surroundings, sights, the sounds, the inner thoughts, feelings, memories, hopes, and dreams, and that's where the attention can be.

Just your feet: mind their business, and you go on your merry way. Hypnosis is a very powerful therapeutic intervention, and you can use it to relax at the same time. The more relaxed you are, the more comfortable you can be.

Dr. Faymonville relaxes people, they relax with her, and they are able to tolerate surgery without an anesthetic. What a wonderful thing that is. So relaxed, so comfortable, and the deeper you go, the more comfortable you can be. Not even knowing how comfortable you are ... more relaxed than you've been for a long... long time.

Being more and more able to find peace and balance, sleep at night feeling whole and loving toward yourself, accepting yourself, nurturing yourself, what a wonderful thing to do, to be r e a l l y ... g o o d ... to ... y o u r s e l f.

In self-hypnosis, when you have ideas they r e a l l y get to percolate, because you can imagine much better in hypnosis, and can imagine being at peace inside yourself, in a way you l o n g e d for, for years and years. And it's there for you. The more relaxed you are, the deeper you can go. Paying attention to the subtle movements and feelings in your body, feeling more and more relaxed!

Colours and thoughts, beautiful sounds, like the breeze in the trees ... the leaves are rustling a soft serenade. The images are there ... the fragrances are there ... the sights are there ... and you can use them to your own satisfaction!

Example Two: Entering another hypnotic trance for my foot pain, with a psychotherapist:

Psychotherapist:

You know the mind is so wonderful in many ways, and one of the nicest ways is to remember pleasures ... You may want to remember what it is like putting your feet in a nice warm bath, or walking along the beach and feeling the sand between your toes, enjoying the waters that ebb up on the beach and cover your feet with a white foamy warm comfortable feeling.

You know, you may remember how cozy it is to have warm socks and warm slippers on, and your feet are nice and warm, just like Goldilocks's porridge, not too hot, not too cold—just right!

You can remember most of your life, not feeling your feet at all, and that wouldn't be a bad thing now, to just let them look after themselves and place your attention on your environment, and watch carefully the clouds drifting by, the sun as it comes down between the limbs of the trees, the pattern of lights in the grass, and you can notice the most subtle changes in people's faces, the beginning of a smile when you tell a joke, and that orthopaedic surgeon who said that he already paid off his mortgage. You know funny expressions ... you become more of your own e x p r e s s i o n s, and less aware of your body at times.

You can remember all the times in your life when you enjoyed hypnosis and relaxing ... You can ask your mind to find its own particular way to bring pleasure, good feelings to those feet, and why shouldn't they feel good?

You may even be able to turn that burning into a warmth, like wearing hot pads and a comfortable warmth at that! I once had a patient who had ringing in his ears, and I found out that he liked opera, so we changed the ringing in the ears to opera music. When you walk the pain goes down, and you can feel the pain getting less and less as time goes by. You become more and more relaxed and focused in other times and other places. Bud, you can ... d r i f t ... easily, comfortably, far, far away, and the comfort spreads throughout your body from the top of your head to the tip of your toes. You don't know how, you don't know why, but somehow your comfort is flowing through your body. It ends up in your feet ... a warm, comfortable, wonderful blue feeling. Blue is cool, and every muscle and every nerve relaxes. You can even hold on to these wonderful, comfortable sensations and ideas as long as you need to, really enjoying all the abilities that you have that can come to the fore ... The deeper you go, the more comfortable you will feel ... and

the more comfortable you are ... the deeper you can go, so easy ....
so comfortable .... take your time .... and just drift ....

Take some time, and more time to relax, knowing that your mind
has many abilities ... some of which you don't know. You know you
that you can go ... far ... far away ... and "*leave your body on a shelf*" so
to speak. ... You can enjoy the soft winds of summer by a lake
somewhere, the lapping of water, and you may even remember
sounds like the loons..... later on the prairies ... in the mornings and
in the evenings ... The sounds that are so... s o o t h i n g ... so ... c o
m f o r t i n g. ... They have been there for many, many generations
... and you can enjoy c o n n e c t i n g with the eternal things ... the
lapping of water ... the shining of the sun ... the softness of a
summer breeze ... the sound of the breeze in the trees. ... In the
evenings... the Milky Way ... things that last forever and a day.

You know the prairies ... the fields of grain, like a sea swaying in the
wind ... the blue, blue sky all around—so relaxing—so peaceful ... and
the deeper you go, Bud, the more comfortable you will be ... The
more comfortable you are, the   d e e p e r you can go. You can go
so deep that you can change the synapses in your mind ... the
comfortable feelings ... all over ... from the top of your head to the
tip of your toes.

When you want to d r i f t ... off ... to ... sleep ... you can pick the
prairie sky—the Milky Way ... and things that last forever and a day
... With each breath, you feel your whole body with interest of ...
relaxation and time ... Time just slows down ... every cell can have a
rest and rejuvenate and heal ... so comfortable. ... You may want to
be more comfortable than you've been for a long, long time ... every
muscle ... every nerve relaxed ... just drifting, far, far away. ... You
can go as far away, Bud, as you need to go ... to find that ultimate
peace ... and be more at peace than you've been for a l o n g, l o n g
time. ... Just enjoy your own ability ... to drift along ... and wander
and wonder ... really relaxed ... every muscle ... every nerve
relaxed...so relaxed. You don't even have to know how relaxed you
are.

*Stan, it has been scientifically established that our bodies react
in the same way to imagined experiences as to real ones. Some*

psychotherapists are using this fact to heal negative childhood experiences.

I, the now adult child, imagine "*going back*" and being a good parent to myself as a child. This therapy can provide the "*self-healing*" of early life traumas of the child who is at last obtaining loving support from his or her self as the original parent.

Example Three: Entering a Hypnotic Trance—"*Going Back*"—Parenting Myself as a Child with a psychotherapist:

"I, big Bud, visualize a lovely image of myself sitting on a park bench during a sunny summer's day as an adult. Then I see "*little Bud*" walking along the path, at age seven. So I, the adult Bud, stopped "*little Bud*" and said, "*Why don't you sit down next to me, and we'll have a little chat.*" I talked to him about this and that and the other, all kinds of things. We laughed, I told him stories, gave him a hug, and added some nurturing things. I told "*little Bud*" that he doesn't have to hold any fears or guilt or shame anymore because I am here and always will be here, to care for and protect "*little Bud*"! Then I gave "*little Bud*" another hug, and felt better myself for doing so."

"We talked for a while, stood up and I took "*little Bud*" by the hand, and we walked to a Dairy Queen, where I bought two Slurpees. We walked, snickered, savoured the scent, sipped, then swilled to empty our containers. We felt so happy, high, dry, and harmonious that we returned to the Dairy Queen for seconds."

"I start a dialogue (so to speak) that I as an adult can protect and nurture the "*little Bud*" aspect of myself through the years. Healing all those experiences that had any negativity in them, being a voice, being comforting with a "*pat on the back,*" being there for a hug, or just smiling, listening, understanding, and I can rewrite my history in a wonderful way, and I can let go of the shame and guilt and negative feelings, and then let go of the letting go, and I just feel free, and the energy comes to me, because all those negative things waste required energy."

"When I let go of the letting go, a boundless and infinite patience, energy, love, and compassion become available for myself. I can even project into the future that adult me, will continue to be there, to heal the parts that need to be healed. I can enjoy the power of my own ability to look into the dark corners and bright light of nurturance, caring for myself, loving myself, being gentle, forgiving, and supportive of myself!!!"

"It is a wonderful metaphor of seeing "*little Bud*" skipping along the path with your adult self there, stopping me and having a little chat about this, that and the other. I can imagine that joy of relaxing deeply, as deeply as I need to go, to enjoy that experience on an experiential power (pertaining to, or derived from experience). I just feel good because I am providing the needs for "*little Bud*" through birthdays, school days, sports days, days where I felt badly because of my older siblings. As a more mature adult, I support and comfort my younger self and my older self too."

"My attitude towards myself becomes a true and trusted friend, and then I realize that I can rely on my unconscious mind, which knows much more than I do, and I can turn my conscious problems over to my unconscious mind for solutions, rewriting history, for doing deep meaningful healing in the past, and going right into the future."

Stan, this is an example of Post-Hypnotic Recall, a true report told to me by the above psychotherapist:

The police visited a tenant in an apartment building because there had been a murder committed next door. This tenant and his wife lived in a fourth-floor apartment, across the hall from the murdered man's suite, so the police asked this couple, "*Did you see any stranger going down the stairs or around this place on Saturday night?*" Neither the husband nor wife could remember any such person.

The psychotherapist put the husband under hypnosis and said to him, "*The mind picks up things that it doesn't even realize. So maybe one morning, you will sit up in bed and you'll realize that you did see somebody that night."*

Several days later, this man returned to see this psychotherapist and stated, *"You know, I sat up in bed about 6:00 o'clock a few mornings ago, and realized that I remembered a man coming down the stairs, as my wife and I went upstairs to the fourth floor, after coming home from a movie."* But he added, *"I can't remember very much detail."*

Then, using a police-hired hypnotist, both the husband and wife were put under hypnotic trances and in separate rooms. A police artist drew a sketch of the stranger's face as the husband recalled seeing the person—first his belt, then his chest, then finally his nose and mouth, eyes and hair. The wife's hypnotic recall description of the stranger matched the description that her husband gave!!!

The detective who interviewed all the suspects, whose names were listed in the murdered man's personal telephone index diary, recognized the artist's drawing as the prime suspect. This detective went to the suspect's home and said, *"We know you did it."*

The suspect was so shocked that he immediately confessed to the murder!

Well, Stan, what do you think of this TRUE, almost incredible, post-hypnotic recall story?

The Conscious and Unconscious Minds by the same psychotherapist:

The conscious mind is that part of the mind that is necessary for survival. It notices the light patterns, the voices, the hum of the refrigerator, the feeling of your body in the chair. Its awareness is diffuse so that you can defend yourself against the unexpected in the environment. It is a diffuse, scattered, vaguely defined awareness.

The unconscious mind is a little bit more than Freud thought it was. The unconscious mind is more than a repository for desires and wants. It also remembers everything that you've ever experienced. And some of the new neuroscience indicates that we know a lot more than we think we know, which Dr. Milton Erickson claimed all the time.

Researchers have proven that this is true by showing slides that move so fast that you don't even know (consciously) that you've seen anything. But the unconscious mind can recognize the difference between angry faces and smiling faces!!! And researchers can tell by looking at PET scans (or using other physiological measures) that even when you don't consciously know you are seeing these things, you can discriminate, even if it's flashed on a screen in a subliminal (subconscious or beneath conscious perception) way.

Your unconscious mind is taking in all kinds of information all the time, and it is a repository of huge amounts of information and knowledge! Often, it's a source of inspiration and creativity beyond the reach of the conscious mind.

Important points to remember about hypnosis:

- All hypnosis is self-hypnosis.
- Suggestions made by a hypnotist under a hypnotic trance will not be accepted unless the person is willing. The person's "*self*" is the controller, not the hypnotist.
- Hypnosis is a relaxed and heightened state of awareness.
- In a trance state, individuals are more susceptible or open to suggestions by the "*self*" via the hypnotist or via self-hypnosis.
- Although usually unaware of it, most people have experienced being in a hypnotic trance; for example, watching a movie or a television program, doing a work project, daydreaming, reading, etc.

An Astonishing Revelation

Stan, while working at the P.N.E., we were given periodic courses in management. The instructor asked us to answer a question on a topic which we studied months ago. I had a two-sentence answer which I had written at that time. Knowing that I had a two-sentence answer for the question, I asked the instructor for a different question. The instructor replied, "There is only ONE question".

Therefore, I began re-writing my two-sentence answer on the topic. Surprisingly, what happened is that my previous short answer was effortlessly expanded to such a degree that it took a long time to complete. Appropriate grammar with persuasive words flowed into my mind with ease and I wrote them down in haste. Now, feeling somewhat guilty about the time I had taken writing and holding up the class, I purposely began to reduce the balance of my text.

Upon completion of my writing, our instructor asked me to read my answer. After I read it, the instructor emphatically replied, *"That was excellent!"* I replied, *"Thank you."*

Later, I overheard our instructor comment to one of our managers, *"If he can write like that, why is he working here?"*

I was also astonished at the amount that I had written with well-suited words, grammar, and without errors. At a much later date, a psychotherapist explained that what I had experienced was called *Automatic Writing.

Automatic writing is the process or product of writing without using the conscious mind. The technique is often practiced while the person writing is in a trance state; others are fully wake, alert, and aware of their surroundings, it is clear that many writers have produced material that they would not have written using only their conscious mind.

*From: http://www.newworldencyclopedia.org/entry/Automatic_writing

Chapter 9 - Meditation

The information below is taken from conversations with a psychotherapist.

Every day we use our brains to think, and rely on our bodies to perform a variety of physical movements. These activities consume energy, and can result in fatigue and emotional stress.

Meditation is a technique that uses your mind to lower the emotional and physical stress levels that have accumulated during the day. By meditating, you can learn to refresh yourself daily, without seeking your sense of value from other people, or depending on drugs and alcohol to feel better. Meditating changes your metabolic rate (the total chemical and physical changes for your body's energy and its functions). And even when you are not meditating, your metabolic system continues to improve, becoming a more efficient system.

Here are some of the proven beneficial effects of meditation. It:

- Lowers heart rate at rest
- Increases peripheral temperature of hands and feet because of easier blood flow
- Increases the release of the hormones serotonin and norepinephrine, resulting in better brain function and lower harmful cortisol secretion
- Lowers blood pressure
- Reduces pain and muscle tension
- Reduces oxygen consumption for specific exercises

- Calms the mind, reduces stress, and relieves anxiety
- Improves concentration and mental clarity
- Improves well-being
- Reduces depression
- Reduces insomnia
- Reduces blood cholesterol
- Reduces the risk of heart attacks

Practising Meditation

Psychotherapist:

For your first meditation, it is best to start in a sitting position with both feet on the floor. At a later date, when you feel up to it, you can meditate while walking, doing tai chi, martial arts, etc.

A lying down position usually promotes sleep while meditating. You do not want meditation to become synonymous with falling asleep. However, lying down to do meditation is acceptable if you have a condition that makes you uncomfortable in a sitting position.

At the beginning, if possible, practise meditation at a set time and in a set location, as free of irritating distractions as possible, with your eyes open or closed as preferred. When you first try meditation, it is good to eliminate visual distractions by keeping your eyes closed.

Now you may place your hands on your abdomen at approximately belt level, with elbows slightly bent and shoulders relaxed. Imagine that you are aware of, or feel, the rise and fall of your hands and belly area with each breath. Also, be aware of the interval between inhaling and exhaling. Take in three consecutive deep breaths without forcing inhalation or exhalation. These breaths provide more oxygen to your blood.

With each breath, concentrate your attention on a word, your breath, or whatever suits you. Slowly, gently, and comfortably inhale through the nose and exhale through your mouth, if possible—whatever works best for you. Feel your breath as it enters with life-supporting air and leaves again. Ideally, be aware of your body, things you are feeling, and accepting the sounds around you.

As your breathing continues, this pattern becomes more spontaneous. By concentrating and being aware of your breathing, you are in the present moment, with awareness only of your breathing and nothing else. If your mind wanders, or if unpleasant or annoying thoughts arise, let them go. Then return to being aware of your breathing as before. By doing so, you train yourself to stop reacting to your stressful thoughts of daily living.

If you feel tensed muscles anywhere, relax them. First, tighten and relax the tensed muscles in a sequence beginning at the toes, then moving to the limbs, stomach, shoulders, arms, neck, chin, forehead, and face. This procedure is known as progressive relaxation.

At the end of your meditation, open your eyes slowly and gently, if closed, then resume your day or night activities. After several successful days of meditating, you may see or feel differences in how you function—perhaps you are less impatient, for example. You can extend these benefits to other activities or situations; for example, when you are sitting in a dentist's chair before you are asked to open your mouth.

For your first meditation attempt, start with about a five-minute session, and gradually increase it by five minutes, ideally to around twenty-minute periods per day making it more effective. Figure out what works best for your schedule.

The more you practise meditation, the better you'll be at keeping cool, calm, and collected. But remember, nobody else can do it for you!!!

If you are anxious about doing meditation correctly, consult someone who has practised it for a long time. Alternatively, read one of many books on meditation at your public library or bookstore, and/or buy some audio meditation tapes. Good relaxed luck!!!

Meditation and Self-hypnosis

Psychotherapist:

Meditation is a tradition of India and Asia, whereas self-hypnosis is more of a Western phenomenon. So, historically, they have different roots. Self-hypnosis has a medical context, with distinct goals of managing symptomatology (the collective symptoms of a patient), and so forth; meditation is more often conducted in spiritual contexts. For example, Buddhism is the most popular context of meditation, with its goal of reaching Nirvana, or becoming at one with your god or universe.

Meditation has a slightly different context, but some people can become quite relaxed with it, just as they can with self-hypnosis, so the end result of both activities is quite similar.

Remember, adequate consistent practice is necessary for both meditation and self-hypnosis if you want to achieve effective results. If you ask somebody to explain what they feel like when they are meditating or practising self-hypnosis, they usually say that everything slows down—their breathing decreases, pulse rate slows down, and all other physiological changes are affected.

Some of the more famous yogis can meditate to the point where they can even stop their hearts for a time! That's how profoundly and intensely they can meditate.

The well-known Dr. Deepak Chopra, when asked what to do about problems that are very difficult to solve, replied: "*Meditate, meditate, meditate*" (source of quote: CNN).

Chapter 10 - Sleep

The information below is taken from conversations with a psychotherapist.

Stan, an adequate sleep period is approximately eight hours. This is the time when our body repairs itself, grows certain tissues, and improves some physiological functions. Body temperature, blood pressure, and breathing rates all decrease during sleep.

Inadequate sleep has a detrimental effect on our immune system which protects us against bacterial, viral, and other foreign substances, and adequate sleep enhances our immune system's performance. During the sleep period, our brain's pea-size pineal gland secretes high amounts of the sleep-enhancer hormone melatonin. Higher stress levels can cause psychosomatic illnesses, and have negative effects on sleep. Our body can learn good or poor sleep patterns.

History

At one time, our distant relatives usually rose at sunrise and went to sleep soon after sunset. Most occupations of that time were physically demanding, and the additional *"workouts"* of today were unheard of—and unnecessary. People in that era followed their rhythmic day/evening life patterns. This was conducive to, and usually allowed for, ample sleep time.

With the advent of the Industrial Revolution, people began to live a more hectic lifestyle. Per capita productivity was dramatically increased, with a parallel increase in the stress levels of society in general. Years later, Edison's electric light bulb invention extended "*daylight*" hours, and so allowed people to go to bed later than they had in the past.

Five Levels of Sleep

1. Transitional or light sleep: a person drifts in and out of sleep.

2. The brain waves slow down and eye movement stops.

3. Slow wave sleep: slow brain waves, or delta waves, occur with faster intermittent small waves, in between slow waves.

4. Almost all brain delta waves are produced. Levels 3 & 4 combined are called deep sleep, or slow wave sleep.

5. Rapid eye movement: REM sleep, or dream sleep, where irregular eye movements occur under closed eyelids. Brain waves increase to awake levels. Muscles are temporarily immobilized. Heart rate and blood pressure both decrease. Men may develop erections. There is some loss of the body's temperature regulation.

During our sleep period, we may cycle through all five levels of sleep several times.

As we age, there is a natural diminishing of the quality and amount of our sleep, but please don't lose any sleep over this!!! It's because the pineal gland, located at the base of the brain, secretes the hormone melatonin, which induces sleep. Slowly, with time, calcium salts are deposited on the pineal gland. These calcium deposits reduce the secretion of melatonin, consequently diminishing our length of sleep time. However, we can improve the quality and amount of our sleep by practising certain skills.

Circadian and Ultradian Rhythms

The circadian rhythm (circa = around + dies = day) pertains to the biological cycles of approximately 24 hours found in animal and plant life. The human circadian rhythm clock is in a group of cells found in the hypothalamus.

Ultradian rhythm is a sleepy lull period, or pattern, which our body goes through about every 90 minutes. It occurs throughout waking and sleeping hours. After approximately 90 minutes, the ultradian rhythm kicks in and lasts for 20 minutes, during which time the brain and body are requesting a natural relaxing break for recuperation. In cases where appropriate breaks are not taken, at about 5:00 pm, for example, people reach a breaking point and become completely exhausted. This is why periodic "*work breaks*" were established.

A power nap, catnap, or siesta is a short sleep, usually 15–30 minutes, during working hours, and is encouraged by progressive companies. Workers become revitalized, especially if they have sleep deficits. The result is fewer employee illnesses and increased productivity.

Tips for Better Sleep

You can retrain your body to give you a better sleep:

- Minimize irritating noises by using foam ear plugs just before going to bed.

- Keep your bed for sleep and sex. Avoid reading, writing, or watching TV while in bed.

- Keep your bedroom dark, or wear a blindfold. Light can disrupt the brain chemicals that regulate sleep.

- If you get up at night, avoid looking at the time. Knowing what time it is can make you more concerned about getting enough sleep, and can cause anxiety and arousal which then further disturbs sleep. If you can't fall asleep after about half an hour, get out of bed and do something.

- Schedule a sleep time, seven days a week!!! Choose the same hour to go to bed every night without much deviation. As soon as you feel sleepy within your bedtime range, "*hit the sack,*" you'll increase your chances of falling asleep. Disrupting your sleep schedule may lead to insomnia, so don't be tempted to sleep late. This will reset your sleep cycle. If you can't fall asleep on schedule, try doing something that is not emotionally stimulating, such as comedy or "*light*" TV (not horror programs!), or reading until you feel drowsy. If you don't feel relaxed enough near bedtime, have a warm bath—but avoid showers, because they are invigorating. A light snack of carbohydrates assists sleep, but do not eat protein. Also, if you go to sleep before your scheduled time, you may wake up too early.

By following the above tips, you will have a good chance of resetting your internal biological clock (circadian rhythm) permanently.

S*tan, it took me quite some time and many, many attempts to "set my clock."*

- If you feel fatigued during the day, limit your nap to about 30 minutes. Long naps can make it more difficult to fall asleep at your scheduled evening time.

- Exercise during the day. Exercise promotes sleep. Exercise no less than six hours before bedtime because exercise too close to your bedtime will delay sleep.

- Keep your bedroom temperature slightly on the cool side for a better sleep.

- Caffeine and nicotine can cause difficulty in falling asleep. Alcohol can help early-stage sleep, but later will cause multiple awakenings.

- If you have a headache or other pain, proper medication will lessen the pain and enhance your sleep.

- Some prescription and over-the-counter medications may contain stimulants that interfere with sleep. Talk to your pharmacist.

- Drinking very little liquids after 6:00 p.m. minimizes waking up during the night to void the bladder.

- When you try very hard to go to sleep, you trigger the negative effect of not going to sleep because you are so "*whipped up*" in trying so hard. And the harder you try, the less likely you are to succeed, because going to sleep is a spontaneous activity, and it is cannot be done on demand!!! So, one way you can get around trying to go to sleep, is by not trying to go to sleep!

- Try hypnosis or mediation. They lead to a very relaxed state of mind with slow breathing and slow heart rate, and to a kind of wandering, wondering mind that leads very naturally to early-phase sleep.

So, part of sleep hygiene is to know how to relax deeply, comfortably, and sink into your mattress. Just let go completely, and then let go of letting go!!!

Chapter 11 - Pain

The information below is taken from conversations with my main psychotherapist.

S *tan, recent studies indicate that 20% of patients suffer from chronic pain. Therefore, I thought we would both be interested in learning more about pain and methods of alleviating it.*

History

Our ancient ancestors thought that pain was caused by demons, and that it could be relieved by professional religious people who used ceremonies and herbs for treatments. Later, Romans, Greeks, and others theorized that the sensation of pain was somehow connected with the nervous system, brain, and spinal cord.

Much later, in the 19th century, physicians found that opium and its derivatives could alleviate pain, but it had side effects such as sleepiness, constipation, and potential addiction. Subsequently, other drugs and anesthetics were developed to relieve pain.

Pain arises from our nervous system and can be described as unpleasant feelings of burning, aching, sharp, dull, tingling, throbbing, searing, nagging, radiating, piercing, intermittent, or constant sensations.

It limits activities because of its physical and psychological impact. Feeling pain, in a sense, is a warning that something is wrong in our body, and we must take action to minimize or stop it, and seek medical advice.

Physical pain has two classes: Neuropathic and Nociceptive.

Neuropathic pain is nerve pain (*neuro* = nerve + *pathos* = suffering). It is also called neurogenic pain (*neuro* = nerve + *genic* = producing). It is a chronic (long-lasting) pain, experienced as burning, tingling, electric-shock-like, or numbing "*going-to-sleep-like*" sensations. Neuropathic pain occurs because of damage to, or dysfunction of, either nerves in the peripheral nervous system (those found outside our brain and spinal cord) or nerves in the central nervous system (those found within our brain and spinal cord).

Types of neuropathic pain:

- Mononeuropathy (*mono* = one) is a disease of a single nerve.
- Polyneuropathy (*poly* = many) is the disease of many nerves.
- Peripheral neuropathy is felt in the extremities such as feet and hands.
- Idiopathic peripheral neuropathy occurs with no apparent or as yet known reason(s).

Some causes and types of neuropathic (i.e. chronic) pain:

- Diabetes can cause diabetic neuropathy.
- Chronic alcohol use can cause widespread peripheral neuropathy.

- HIV/AIDS and their medications can cause peripheral neuropathy.
- Thyroid problems, e.g., a bacterial infection called acute thyroiditis.
- Shingles is caused by the chickenpox virus Herpes Zoster. It may affect nerves in the face, chest, or abdomen, usually with painful skin blisters. The pain may be severe and last a few weeks or up to several months.
- Vitamin B1, B6, B12, E, niacin, and zinc deficiencies may result in neuropathic pain.
- Toxins, such as arsenic, lead, and certain chemotherapies, may cause neuropathic pain.
- Neuralgia is a severe nerve pain. A stabbing or burning pain after shingles. Another type is in the face, which can occur on successive days.
- Nerve damage after an injury heals. Sometimes nerve damage results from surgery.
- Post-limb-amputation. Where nerve damage occurs during surgery. The limb is severed but there is a sensation that the limb, or part of it, is still attached, called phantom limb pain.
- Fibromyalgia is the pain felt in muscles and their tendons and ligaments. Its exact cause is not yet known. It is currently suspected that emotional stress, infection, and physical injuries may be contributing factors.
- Irritable bowel syndrome. This condition may be caused by anxiety, emotional stress, or intestinal infection. The result is pain, constipation, and diarrhea. (Note: There is a huge controversy about whether or not fibromyalgia and irritable bowel syndrome are in the neuropathic pain category.)

- Carpal tunnel syndrome. This condition occurs when a compressed nerve in the wrist enters the palm of the hand. The result causes numbness and pain in the fingers.
- Spinal cord injuries; e.g., fractured vertebrae, herniated discs.

Neuropathic pain treatments:

- Analgesics are both narcotic and non-narcotic. Non-narcotics used are usually acetaminophen (Tylenol), ibuprofen, Aspirin. They are used for low to moderate pain relief. Neuropathic pain is usually not relieved with these over-the-counter medications.
- Narcotic analgesics are the most potent pain relievers, but they have undesirable side effects such as sleepiness, constipation, and possible addiction. Two opium derivatives are codeine and morphine.
- Diabetics who keep their blood sugar under control will reduce their peripheral neuropathic pain.
- Diabetics who monitor their blood sugar levels can control these high levels with medications and exercise. Diabetics can use sucrose for low blood sugar levels to reduce their neuropathic pain.
- Cortisone compounds and anesthetics are sometimes used to alleviate neuropathic pain.
- Antidepressants in small doses are used to alleviate chronic pain and assist sleep.
- Anticonvulsants, such as Lyrica, Gabapentin, Topamax, Tegretol.
- Non-analgesics neuropathic pain relievers:
    - Warm or cold compresses, warm baths/foot baths.

o Acupuncture or acupressure.

o Hypnosis and meditation can relax a person, lower stress, and can alleviate neuropathic pain.

o Physiotherapy exercises.

o TENS units give electrical impulses to nerves in the pain area.

o Massage therapy on aching body areas.

Nociceptive pain (from *noci* = injury or pain + to receive) refers to nerve fibre endings and/or pathways concerning pain. Nociceptors are unique nerve endings that were discovered in 1906 by Charles Sherington. Nociceptor receptors are found throughout our body. Nociceptor nerve endings are clever: they react only to potentially damaging pain stimuli, and not to other normal stimuli such as touching.

Nociceptive pain is generally caused by damaged tissue. It is not caused by damaged nerves like neuropathic pain. It is felt as aching, burning, bruising, throbbing, dull, or sharp, and is sometimes accompanied by neuropathic pain.

Nociceptors are triggered by three pain patterns:

11. Mechanical pain, as in a broken bone.

12. Ischemic pain, or the blockage or constriction of a blood vessel (e.g., when there is constriction of a blood vessel in the heart resulting in angina pectoris pain).

13. Inflammation pain, or the reaction of tissue to injury. It may be caused by bacterial/viral infections. Blood vessels at the site dilate to increase blood flow. Blood components engulf foreign particles and bacteria. Cells of similar nature consume and remove dead cells

causing pus formation, thus encouraging the healing process.

Some causes of nociceptive pain:

- Inflammation.
- Cuts, surgery.
- Burns
- Bruises.
- Cold.
- Extreme pressure.

Nociceptive pain has two subtypes:

1. Somatic pain.

- Somatic pain is felt in the outer parts of the body in bone, bone joints, muscle, ligament, and tendon injuries. Joint pain is called musculoskeletal pain. The sex organs are not included. Somatic pain is well localized and constant. The peripheral nervous system carries these pain sensations.
- External nociceptor receptors are located on the skin, cornea of the eyes, etc.
- Somatic pain examples include multiple sclerosis and arthritis.

2. Visceral pain.

- Visceral pain is felt in the internal organs such as the stomach, intestines, lungs, kidneys, etc.
- Visceral pain is poorly localized. Pain is intermittent within internal organs such as with gall bladder stones.
- Internal nociceptors are in body organs, such as the liver, muscles, joints, stomach, etc. The central nervous system carries these pain sensations.

- Visceral pain examples include stomach ulcer pain, cancer pain, porphyria, and angina.

Nociceptors, when triggered, transmit:

- Afferent impulses (carried toward the brain), regulated by neurotransmitters through the peripheral nervous system (PNS) to the spinal cord, then into our brain's thalamus and cerebral cortex for processing. This information then becomes our conscious awareness of pain, as well as non-painful sensations of touch, temperature, etc.

- Efferent impulses (carried away from the brain), regulated by neurotransmitters released from the hypothalamus to reduce pain sensation. This is how the somatic signal loop is completed. The visceral nociceptive signal loop follows this pattern, but through the central nervous system (CNS).

- Acute pain (*acutus* = rapid onset). This pain begins suddenly, may be of severe intensity, and is of relatively short duration. It may be caused by injuries to body tissue, such as cuts and bruises. Other acute pains are felt as headaches, muscle cramps, intestinal gas bloating, or toothaches, and in sinuses. Acute pain may cause shock, or increases in blood pressure, breathing, and heart rate. Nociceptive pain is acute. It lasts for a relatively short period of time because the tissue damage has healing potential. Arthritis is one exception because it does not have this healing advantage.

- Chronic pain (*chronos* = time). Chronic pain lasts a long time (more than six months), and it sets in gradually. It may be severe to moderate in intensity, and is very difficult to eliminate. Neuropathic pain is chronic, lasting indefinitely because the nerves in neuropathy are affected in ways that healing them has yet to be discovered. However, neuropathic pain can be alleviated. Chronic pain may also begin as a gradual onset of acute pain. Some examples of chronic pain are arthritis, damaged nerves, cancer, back pain, and headaches.

Stan, I am reducing my chronic pain with medication and exercise. Some people can endure pain without pain medication. Other people depend only on pain medication to relieve it. Such people favour their chronic pain area, and make little or no effort to move or use it for fear of making their pain condition worse. Stan, I was in this category for some time, "losing it by not using it," and making my neuropathic foot pain worse!

Atrophy of muscles, in one or more parts of our body, occurs through disuse and aging. Adequate prescribed exercises keep muscles toned.

I consulted a physician at a pain clinic about combining pain medication and exercise. His reply was positive. He exercises five days a week, taking a small amount of pain medication, plus another medication for his diabetes!

Now I am taking prescribed pain medication for my condition, which reduces the pain to a tolerable level so that I am able to cope with several physiotherapy exercises for my neuropathic foot pain.

I have begun to walk more. The walking distance is dependent on the level of my foot pain.

After a physician checks out the nature of a patient's pain disorder, he or she may employ additional methods to determine the exact origin of the pain. Blood tests and specialized equipment may also be used as follows:

- Bone imaging: This is a technique for diagnosing bone fractures and other bone disorders, and to monitor infections. A tiny amount of radioactive substance is injected into the patient's bloodstream. The radioactive material gathers in abnormal bone areas. The scanned images are sent to a computer to show specific abnormal bone areas, and normal or abnormal blood flow. This diagnostic procedure gives a more accurate and detailed diagnosis of most bone disorders.

- Computed tomography (CT or CAT scan): "*Tomography*" comes from the Greek tomos = slice + graphein = to write. X-rays and computers are used to give a cross-section of a patient's body. A blood test may be taken prior to the scan. A contrast material is injected into the patient's vein and the patient, lying on a table, is told to stay as still as possible. The table is then moved through a large "*hole-in-a-doughnut*" scanning device. This diagnostic procedure may last from several minutes to an hour.

- Discography: This diagnostic technique uses a special dye that is injected into a patient's problem spinal disc to show x-ray contrast. An x-ray picture is taken of the spinal disc(s) thought to be causing the back pain. The disc(s) may or may not show tears in the disc's lining. Depending on the results, surgery or another treatment is carried out.

- Electromyography or EMG: This diagnostic procedure uses fine needles that are inserted into muscles to measure their electrical response (while contracting and at rest) from the brain and/or spinal cord.

- Magnetic resonance imaging (MRI): This diagnostic procedure, first used in 1977, uses a computer, radio waves, and large magnet to produce detailed images with greater contrast between soft body tissues than those produced by CAT scans. It is best used for cancer, cardiovascular, musculoskeletal, brain, and neurological imaging. (People with any metallic (knee) implants, or pacemakers, should avoid having MRI tests.)

- Ultrasound or diagnostic sonography: this uses high-frequency sound waves emitted from a hand-held device, which is placed on and moved across a patient. A water gel transfers the sound vibrations from the hand-held device to the patient. It is used for imaging soft tissues, such as kidneys, livers, foetuses, breasts, testicles, tendons, ligaments, and muscles.

- Myelograms or myelography: A form of x-ray called fluoroscopy. A contrast dye is injected into the spinal canal to give better x-ray images. The injected dye causes pain in the spinal canal. Myelograms are currently falling out of favour.

Psychogenic pain

Psychogenic (from the Greek *psycho* = mind + *genic* = origin) pain originates in the mind, because of some current or extended unexpressed emotional conflicts. There is no evidence of tissue or any other physical damage caused by psychogenic pain. Certain emotional conditions that cause psychogenic pain influence its severity and duration. Psychogenic pain is usually chronic, and feels like physical pain.

Some chronic psychogenic pain examples:

- Muscle pain.
- Headaches.
- Stomach pain.
- Back pain.

Acute psychogenic pain is caused by what a person sees, or feels, as problems of the more recent past and as future difficulties. Symptoms may include:

- Sweaty and/or cold hands and feet.
- Heartburn.
- Constipation or diarrhea.
- Intestinal gas.
- Tension or migraine headaches.
- Painful esophageal spasms.
- Emotional upsets.
- Anxiety and depression.
- Heart palpitations.
- Hypertension.
- Episodes of worry and rushing.

Acute psychogenic pain can be treated with quality psychotherapy and prescribed medications.

Causes of psychogenic pain

Stress is a normal response to the expected pressures we face in life. However, if a person finds it a more fearful struggle to control such pressures, a build-up of stress occurs, and if continued, can result in adverse effects. When a person has a fearfully high stress response, the brain's hypothalamus triggers an alarm, causing an overdose of the stress hormones cortisol and adrenaline.

Adrenaline increases blood pressure/heart rate and cortisol suppresses growth, the digestive system, and the immune system.

Such a person is at risk of:

- Slowing down the body's repair rate.
- Heart disease.
- Insomnia.
- Indigestion.
- Suppressing the immune system.
- Memory impairment.
- Emotional disorders: anger, anxiety, depression.
- Gastrointestinal disorders: bloating, diarrhea, nausea.
- Pain symptoms in the chest, extremities, head, back, joints.
- Irregular menstruation.
- Excessive bleeding during menstruation.
- Sexual dysfunction.
- Erectile dysfunction.
- Psychosocial disorders.

Acute psychogenic pain can be treated with high-quality psychotherapy and prescribed medications.

Chronic psychogenic pain often develops in people who come from dysfunctional families:

- They have had shocking childhood experiences.
- These experiences are learned very early in life, so they live under a "*cloud*" of almost continual fear.
- These negative feelings require long-term psychiatric treatment because the thoughts are difficult, but not impossible to erase.

Chronic depression:

- Can be caused by many factors such as a chemical imbalance of the important neurotransmitters, dopamine, norepinephrine, and serotonin, which help the neurons in the brain communicate with each other.
- May also be caused by genes and/or the pain of chronic negative thoughts. Such stressful thinking wears down the body.

Chronically stressed people may suffer from heart disease or strokes, or even become suicidal.

Chapter 12 - R is for Remembering,

Including a few repetitions of the previous most tormenting experiences, plus input from one psychotherapist.

R1. One of the first moments I can recall is me lying in my crib. One of several family members who stood around the crib anchored a new multicoloured toy above me. I reached up with one hand and turned a red coloured wheel on the toy. I did not find it very interesting. Some of these family members made some comments and walked away, leaving me alone. I felt abandoned, not part of *"the pack."* I wanted to be with them. My only comfort was to look at the toy or the embossed pattern on the ceiling.

Stan, how do you think I would have felt if a smiling family member had picked me up out of the crib, held me close in his or her arms, and taken me into the kitchen with the rest of the family—happier, comforted, and at ease?

I did not feel a daily connection to my family members. I felt somewhat neglected and unknown because of not receiving adequate comfort from parents and siblings. At this early age, the lack of a supportive, nurturing environment began to put me at risk of depressive disorders. Later, when I was able to stand up in my crib, I looked out through the bedroom doorway for some companionship, which seemed slow to arrive. I felt very lonely.

Even now, when I find myself alone for several hours I slide into an uncomfortable mood, feeling insecure, isolated, and deserted until I phone someone, or my wife comes home.

Psychotherapist:

As you say, you slide into an uncomfortable mood, feeling insecure, isolated, and deserted, until you phone someone, or your wife comes home.

One of the things that strikes me about that, Bud, is that I was reading that people who have been abused as kids develop this similar pattern of feelings, negative feelings that stem from early days. They are talking about (this was on the Deepak Chopra Show actually) a lot of the kids who have been abused. It appears that 25% of that population has suffered some form of abuse.

That 25%, when you watch them through the years, with regard to autoimmune disease, such as lupus, scleroderma, arthritis, sjogren's syndrome, and the like, they are over-represented in that group. In other words, you are vulnerable for illness if you had abuse problems as a kid.

We often talked about sibling abuse, and to some extent, parental abuse of yourself and that has haunted you through your life. Then, how do you manage negative feelings?

We talked a lot about letting go, and moving on, because those negative feelings, caused by other people, if we hold onto them, then we are not living up to our own responsibility of actual forgiveness and forgetting, and "move-on scenario," because we are ultimately responsible for our inner peace. If you want your inner peace to grow, you have to settle all the accounts outstanding. Sometimes the only way to settle them is to forgive the offender and even treat the offender well with no explanation! Guilt is a negative emotion, and if you are trying to make the cup half empty, any little negative emotion can cause it!!!

In reality, pain is part of life. Forgiveness allows you to let go of that negative part, so you don't have to carry around that bitterness, they were wrong and you were right. But you can get beyond right and wrong, who is right and who is wrong!!!

Now, especially now, in your later years, so you can enjoy friends, and your day-to-day mundane life, and not so mundane when you are not carrying around a load of negativity!

Going back to R1, you can get into the habit of thinking negatively when you are alone, so when you are alone, and you start to drift in that direction, go after your tapes, Bud, and rewrite or rewire your brain so that alone means time for inner peace, and tranquility, and exploration, and contemplation, so that you change the whole paradigm of being alone, as something to look forward to!

Part of the negativity, of course, is fear! A sense of security is what battles fear, a sense of faith in yourself, belief in yourself! Whatever other people say, *"Sticks and stones will break my bones, but names will never hurt me"*!!!

Stan, this statement is likely true for many people, and being called "Asshole" and "Booby" by my two brothers and their friends did much to lower my self-esteem in the past, but now, at last, I am beginning to forgive them, and forget those ugly, degrading names of the past!!!

R2. I remember one day when my mother changed my diaper. There was a pleasant smile on her face. A blue, pink, and white-coloured can of baby powder stood on my left. When the diaper was pinned together I felt warmer, smiled, and felt connected with my mother—an example of good nurturing. I was in a happy frame of mind on these occasions.

R3. While being moved around in a carriage, at times I wore a maroon-coloured wool pullover sweater. When my mother decided that I was too warm, she pulled it off. I recall the sweater being removed, because the rough wool irritated my face and I would give out a cry of protest.

R4. While sitting on my mother's knee being fed, I remember not wanting to swallow the food in my mouth. I don't know how my mother knew, but she put her hand to my mouth and I spit it out, the food contained a fishbone!

R5. I recall my mother and a family member beckoning me to walk. I took one step forward and fell. Then I stood up, and took a few steps to reach them.

R6. One evening I was in bed with my parents, and I was breastfeeding. I did not understand what my father said to my mother, but his tone of voice and inflection suggested to me that he was complaining, *"How much longer will he be breastfeeding?"*

I did not have a monopoly, and I was willing to share, because there was room for two. I felt shamed, thinking that I had done something *"wrong."* This painful *"put-down"* helped to lower my self-esteem to such an extent that I promptly stopped breastfeeding on my 15th birthday.

That last part was a joke, Stan!

R7. While in my high chair, I watched and listened to my parents, who were sitting across from each other at the kitchen table. I had the best seat in the house, the high chair. I did not understand what they were discussing but their voices were loud and angry. I did not know why they were so upset, but I was not a happy camper. I was startled and bewildered by these frequent *"discussions,"* and frightened by my father's very loud voice. When the arguments ended, my father left through the back door, slamming it shut. For me, these traumatic experiences put me firmly on the path of becoming fearful!

R8. When I was quite young, I contracted pertussis (whooping cough). My coughing eventually caused a left inguinal hernia. As a result, I remember wearing a truss that was strapped at the hernia level and pressed against the abdominal bulge. In time the hernia seemed to recede, but many years later, when an adult, two inguinal hernias developed which were corrected by surgery.

R9. At about age three, I was shown how to draw with pencil and paper. I was drawing a picture of a sailing ship which was featured on the cover of an Eaton's catalogue. My older sister Tory was showing me how to draw waves around the ship. My father came along to take a look at the drawing. When he saw me drawing with my left hand, he ordered me, in a loud, commanding voice, to draw using my right hand. He did not have to order me to do so a second time: I switched to my right hand in a flash. I had been afraid of him for quite some time. I felt guilty for doing something wrong. This was a negative thought that undermined my self-confidence and increased my potential for depression.

R10. I remember my toilet training. As I sat on the toilet completing my bowel movement, my mother would, too often, watch me through the partly open bathroom door with a smiling face. This smile is one that I always associated with ridicule. I felt embarrassed even though I passed the "drop test" with flying colours. Years later, I realized that my mother's observation of me during those few minutes made me feel shamed for lack of privacy, even though she did everything correctly.

R11. Before I attended school, my two brothers and two sisters would come home from school for the one-hour lunch break. Soon after we finished most of our lunch, tea was served. While my mother was out of sight in the kitchen, my brother Ted poured tea for my sister Vera. Vera raised her cup for Ted to pour the tea into it. Ted purposely poured hot tea on Vera's hand. Vera screamed in pain and our mother ran into the dining room to find out what had happened. Then Ted told our mother that Vera had moved her hand into the stream of hot tea. For whatever reasons, Ted seemed to dislike Vera.

R12. Once before my birthday, I was very happy about getting older. I ran out into the front yard hollering, "*I'll be four years old on May the fourth.*" A neighbour Olga, walking by stopped to ask me about the other months. The only one I was aware of was the month of May. I was somewhat disappointed in not knowing names of the other months, then Olga told me that the next month was June.

R13. I watched my mother using an electric curling iron on her hair. I was very interested in how the curling iron created the hair curls. When my mother finished using the iron, she placed it on the kitchen table, and probably warned me that it was hot. If I did get a warning, I did not heed it. When my mother left the kitchen, I climbed up on a chair next to the table, and then onto the table itself. I got close to the hot iron, and reached out to touch it with my index finger of my right hand. The iron was hot enough to make a burn just below the fingernail, which left a permanent visible scar. I cried out in pain with tears running down my cheeks. When I looked up, I saw my mother walk into the kitchen with a broad smile. With me in pain, and my mother smiling, I did not feel comforted even though I was at fault for touching the hot curling iron. Her reaction to this traumatic event, I thought, revealed little compassion.

R14. Our mother went to Winnipeg one day to do some shopping and visiting. On that day, my brother Ted had to look after me and my sister Vera. We spent much of the day in the basement, where Ted was working on a project. Ted was the *"Mr. Fix-It"* in our family. Ted decided to smoke a cigarette while we were in the basement, and he cautioned me not to mention this to Mom. Naturally, being supportive of my *"big brother,"* I agreed not to tell her. When Mom came home, I remember walking up the basement steps with Ted and Vera. As I promised Ted, I did not tell Mom that he had been smoking. Thinking that I was reinforcing Ted's smoking secret, the first thing I said to her was, *"Mom, Ted was not smoking, honest!"*

R15. I was aware that, not yet old enough to attend school, I was the only one who could not read in our family of seven. Therefore, I decided to learn to read by looking at books. I sat on the floor in front of the bookcase, and looked at books literally for hours on end. One book was called The Doctor's Book, and contained lift-up coloured drawings of human organs. I was careful not to pull off these cut-outs. However, my mother felt that this *"medical reference book"* was in peril, and took it out of my lap and placed it out of my reach. Most of the books were printed in English, but some were printed in Ukrainian Cyrillic script. I noticed the difference, which only made my reading quest a deeper mystery. After what seemed like ages, I thought that I had finally "*cracked the reading code.*" Upon looking at a book in Cyrillic script, I noticed that one of the letters appeared to me at least, to be a "*symbol*" for a wood and coal-fired space heater. I ran to my mother with the book, and asked her if the letter meant "*heater.*" My mother smiled and said no. She added that in order to learn how to read, I would have to wait until I was old enough to begin school at age six. This reply dashed my hopes for learning how to read, leaving me sad and perhaps was the beginning of my depression. No one in the family offered to teach me how to read.

R16. One day the whole family drove to a Winnipeg Park for a picnic. After lunch, I was taken to see some animals. Near a wire mesh fence, I was given some food in my hand and told to feed an animal. At four years of age, I was very close to the ground. All that my eyes were fixed on was something sliding back and forth against the fence and grass. I had no idea what the "*thing*" was until much later. I was scared stiff as family members encouraged me to hand "*it*" the food. After this frightening event, I was told that what I had been frightened by was an animal's huge tongue moving back and forth.

R17. Occasionally we visited the Boheme family on their farm in St. Anne, Manitoba, my birthplace. They had a large family with a small daughter about my age. Often during these visits, I was hoisted up on the back of one of the Boheme sons to carry me across a stream, to go to pick wild berries.

Once, just before our visit ended, I was presented with a gift. The gift was a little cock, or rooster, named Peteyou. I was very happy with Peteyou who was never aggressive towards me. Peteyou seemed happy, especially when I fed and played with him each day. One day after dinner, I went out to the backyard and called for Peteyou. He usually came running to me, but now he was nowhere in sight. I ran back into the house and alerted the family that Peteyou was gone. I cannot recall what reasons were given for his absence, but the family members did not seem alarmed that he was not around. Years later, I found out that Peteyou, the cock, had been castrated and then called a capon. The de-sexing of Peteyou was said to improve the flavour of the flesh when used as food. And so, unknown to me at the time, poor Peteyou would never hear me again, because he, or what was left of him, lay motionless on the kitchen table. This was a painful loss for me.

R18. One of my playmates, named Metro, lived about a city block from me. Once we found two dead sparrows in Metro's front yard. We decided to bury the birds after lunch. I went home and asked my mother why they had died, and whatever the answer was, I felt bewildered and sad.

Metro's Uncle Max drove a bakery delivery truck and visited Metro's parents frequently. Metro knew his uncle's schedule, and at the appropriate time we would hide in Shaw's *"vacant haunted house"* directly across the street. After Uncle Max was seen entering Metro's house, Metro and I would go to the rear of the truck, and Metro opened the back door and entered. I served as the lookout. Metro was quick to pick up some goodies, and we both made tracks for the veranda of the *"haunted house."* The shortbread was always fresh and tasty.

R19. When I was only a few years old, a friendly neighbour named Barney took me by the hand, and walked me for about one city block to their empty cow barn. Their cows were out to pasture. Barney took me to the far end of the unlit barn and left me there. As he walked away he said to me, *"Now the cows will come in and get you!"* I stood petrified and crying, fearing the entrance of cows at any moment. Eventually I stopped crying. I walked along the dark side of the wall with the open door. As I walked towards the light of the open door, I was in constant fear that the cows would come in, blocking my path before I could walk out to freedom. This very frightening event increased my level of fear!

R20. Having a tricycle, I had to shop at Polny's corner grocery store, approximately one city block away from home. On the way to Polny's, I had to pass Petri's angry dog twice. I was afraid of this dog even though it was fenced in. While passing this barking dog, I could see between spaces in the picket fence, its open mouth with large teeth and dripping saliva. This repeated scene for me, at such an early age, was a terrifying, long-lasting memory! Later, Petri's dog bit two neighbours. I was told that the police were advised, and the dog was shot while it was still in the owner's yard.

R21. Two neighbourhood sisters often came over to our house to play with my sister Vera and me. The older girl, Evy, was about my sister Vera's age, and the younger sister, was my age. One day we went upstairs and I picked up an alarm clock which we thought did not work. The clock started ticking. Vera and Evy, happily hollered to my mother that I had fixed the clock. I noticed soon after, that the clock stopped ticking. It wasn't fixed!

R22. While Vera and Evy were at school, Nora would sometimes come over to play. When Nora's mother came to pick up her daughter at lunchtime, both our mothers spoke Ukrainian to each other. Although I did not understand that language well, I could sense through non-verbal communication that their almost convulsive laughter was directed at Nora and me, just for being playmates. A psychotherapist once told me that "*being laughed at is a major insult*," and I agree.

Beginning from that time, and for well over ten consecutive years thereafter, my mother and older sister Tory (Victoria) teased me about having Nora, a girl, as a playmate!

Both my mother and Tory would mention the name Nora, always with a grin, then watch me react as I turned to walk away, cringing in corrosive shame. My mother and Tory received their sadistic pleasure by "*teasing me*" for having a female childhood playmate. Was this sadistic verbal abuse? I took it as such. Their "*teasing*," or "*just kidding*," did not make me become "*femaphobic*" or "*gay*," just very unhappy!

This sadistic teasing made me feel like avoiding the companionship of females, even though this natural desire was well established in me. I actually felt that I had no control over this natural inherent need. I was shamed out of this normal "*male attraction to females*," and this shame undermined my self-confidence, another step towards depressing my frame of mind.

Psychotherapist:

What is teasing? Teasing often has a "*barb*" in it or a "*hook*," and again, it's a sort of "*power move*" on the part of "*the teasers*" to feel better. If the object of the "*teasing*" is embarrassed and hurt, then, they feel more powerful!!! Teasing, I've read about, is a form of, just as you say, Bud, sadism!!!

Again, teasing is how to make the teaser feel better! Teasing is an insecurity operation in the sense that "*teasers*" need to stand on other people's shoulders to feel better!!!

I had my first date, away from home, when I was 23 years old! In view of the above-mentioned "*teasing*" or "*bullying*," I felt that if I ever made a woman pregnant, I would have to legally change my name and move to a different location.

Stan, that is how shamed I felt!!!

R23. The shaming that I received from my mother and sister Tory when they mentioned the name Nora left an indelible mark in my mind. In later years, whenever I passed Nora's mother and older sister, Evy, on the street, my eyes looked downward, because I was too ashamed even to say "*Hello*" to them. I felt guilty!!!

Psychotherapist:

Okay, Bud, sit back, relax, and enjoy being "*mesmerized*" like your sister said.

As you noted, you were shamed when you were just a little kid, which can be a searing experience as you say, and especially when it comes from your mom and your older sister who are supposed to love you, right? On top of that it is sort of a normal thing for a four or five year old to hang out together. My sister, when she was about four or five, had a little baby carriage, and placed the neighbour's dog in it, on its back, pretending that it was a baby. The little dog was named Paddy. So we had quite the gang of kids and it was quite pleasant, total normal activities.

So why your mom and older sister would pick on you is a mystery. Somehow you would like to let go of that shame, that fear, that hurt, that pain. You can, Bud, because the human mind is resilient, you know. So when you get those memories, you can start to put them in perspective that it is a normal thing for kids to play together in that age group.

It's a wonderful thing that black kids, yellow kids, and white kids all play together, they don't know about colour discrimination. There is something very innocent and wonderful about kids connecting just intuitively.

So there is nothing wrong with you Bud, there is nothing wrong with the little girl. What the problem is are the adults like your mother and sister. What is called "a cheap thing," they were raising their self-esteem by being critical of you and the girl, as if to say they are superior in some way. So maybe you can forgive them because it's a sad thing that they have to use that kind of way to feel better about themselves. That is to say, when they can accuse or blame or run down somebody else, then that makes them feel powerful and strong. This negative attitude is what I call "a cheap way," especially when kids are involved.

You hear of some bosses who do it to their employees, especially their secretaries, the vulnerable ones. I had a secretary as a patient, Bud, who had a boss who was miserable like that. Every time she tried to tell him off she started crying. So I sent her to assertiveness classes and she was able to role play her boss with other people who took the boss's grumpy attitude. Finally she went to her boss's office. She told him off and said that not only should you stop bullying I've also copied my thoughts to the president of the company. Also, I did mention to the president that you've had 10 secretaries in the last three years and this is the kind of thing you are doing to them. So that boss was fired by the president of the firm, so he got his comeuppance.

So if you can imagine, Bud, you can play that scenario over again in your mind's eye and stand up to your mother and sister by saying, *"Look, this is a normal activity, smarten up and don't raise your self-esteem in that kind of 'cheap way."* So you can play that scene, Bud, and it will probably realign your circuits, to use a metaphor, in your mind. You can go back in time and coach that four-year-old Bud to stand up to his mother and sister.

Remember the movie Christmas Carol with Scrooge in it? The Ghost of Christmas Past took him back into the past, which had a look at things, and then he was able to alter them in his mind to put them into the right place. Then, remember, Scrooge went over to his nephew's place and started dancing because he thought that he had let his sister down because she died giving birth to her son, which was his nephew. I watch that movie every year and it makes me cry it's so moving.

You can rewrite your story, Bud, the way you want it to be. Then in your rewriting, your editing, you might say to your mom and your sister, *"Look here now, I'm only four but I know better than you."*

It's a normal thing for a four-year-old to play together with peers. It's a wonderful thing in fact for kids not to know that sex matters or colour matters or where they come from matters, just two little kids naturally playing in a wonderful way, so you can rewrite your history, Bud, and this is the way to do it. So you can go now as deeply as.. you.. need.. to.. for.. a.. minute.. or.. so.. and s....l.....o.....w.....l.....y .....let yourself ...come... back... to... the... here... and... now.

R24. I must have taken a page out of their sadistic book. I overheard that a neighbour named Stanley had a girlfriend. Stanley passed our house regularly, on his way to work. Whenever I saw Stanley passing by, while I was in the front yard, what did I say? *"Stanley has got a girlfriend, Stanley has got a girlfriend,"* on and on. Stanley seemed to be annoyed at what I kept teasing him about. One day Stanley met my brother Joe, and told him what I was constantly saying to him. Then, in my presence, Joe came into the house in anger, and told our mother what I kept saying to Stanley, adding, "*You know, Stanley is twenty-seven years old.*" One scowling look from my mother was enough to stop me from teasing Stanley. So mom and Tory had "*the green light*" to tease me, but I was given "*the red light*" not to tease— a double standard that I did not quite understand.

R25. One method my mother had for keeping me in line, if my behaviour was unacceptable, was the frightening threat of Mr. Skinner. If I did not stop misbehaving, my mother threatened to call Mr. Skinner. Mr. Skinner would then come to our house and, in her words, "*Skin me alive!!!*"

Stan, at that age I believed that this was a valid threat that would likely cause my painful death! So I tried not to misbehave, and never did see Mr. Skinner!

Psychotherapist:
And when your mother was talking about "*Mr. Skinner*" you were vulnerable, and now you can go back to that little boy, and see him come up and sit beside you on the park bench. And he sees you there reading a paper. Eventually, he'll ask you what you are going to do, and you'll say, "*I'm going to drive my car, but I can't get out of the garage, because the door is shut.*" So then, Bud, you realize that there is an opener to the door, and doors do open for you. You feel more free to do your own thing, and fear begins to go away when you have a goal, a passion, a drive. LOVE gives you energy, and you can find a place where love is.

LOVE melts away fear, especially love of yourself. LOVE towards your mother, knowing that she probably did the best she could, under her world view, or her circumstances. Then the other thing is, that "*Mr. Skinner*" never came over to your house, so when it comes to fear, there are many "*paper tigers*" out there!!!

So many years later, thanks to my psychotherapist, I have a better understanding of my frightened childhood experiences, and finally, I'm on the road to forgiveness and forgetting!!!

R26. My mother told me that I was not to be friendly with, or play with, Ernie, a neighbourhood boy. The reason for avoiding Ernie was that his mother had been divorced, and later remarried. The divorce and remarriage had turned poor Ernie into a stepson. My mother obeyed the Catholic decree, which supported one marriage without divorce. Not knowing any better, I sometimes disobeyed my mother and went to play with Ernie.

R27. At times, when I was very young, I would sit on the floor of our front veranda and watch the smoke coming out of a tall chimney located some distance away in the Canadian National Railway Shops. I wondered why the smoke seemed to *"disappear"* when it was not far from the smokestack. Another mystery was lightning. I sat in the same place on the front veranda, watching lightning in the sky. I was fascinated by the different streaks of lightning. Every flash of lightning seemed to have a different shape. Once during my *"observations"* nobody in the family could find me. Then my mother, with an alarmed look on her face, opened the screen door, came over, and quickly picked me up and took me into the safety of the house.

R28. I must have seen bigger boys doing something skillful, and began to try it myself. I climbed up on the front yard picket fence, and started walking and balancing myself on the top two-by-four. As I progressed along the fence, my mother happened to come out of the front door, and she fearfully hollered my name. I jumped off the fence, traumatized, as soon as I heard the scream. I never attempted that feat again. However, I did try to climb a front yard tree, but I was too short at the time to reach the lower branch.

R29. One time Vera took me to Evy's house, halfway up the block. Several children were playing in the area. In the front yard we saw small white butterflies flying around. I was warned by some of the children to avoid the white butterflies because if one landed on my face it would sew my mouth shut, and then I would not be able to eat or talk. Well, I was scared stiff of those butterflies. When I arrived home, I asked my mother if the white butterflies really would sew my mouth shut. My mother told me that they would not sew my mouth shut. However, even after having the truth explained to me, the fear had a hold on me, and I kept avoiding the white butterflies.

R30. I saw the older boys with whom my two older brothers kept company. They usually grouped together halfway down the block, on the opposite side of the street from our house. Once in a while I went over to hear what the group had to say. On one particular day, I heard three words that were new to me.

I went home and proudly told my mother the three words that I had just added to my vocabulary, "*God damn it.*" My mother said not to repeat those words again because they were very bad words. I agreed, and then said, "*I will never say God damn it, again because God damn it is not nice to say.*" So even though I now knew not to say these three new bad words, I did get a kick out of repeating them.

R31. There were many instances where what I said to my mother must have been a stretch of my imagination, or outright lies. My mother often caught me distorting the truth, and I began to think she knew I was going to lie as soon as I began to speak. Mom then said to me, although not in anger, "*You little lallu*" (liar). I didn't enjoy being caught lying. Eventually, I got my mom's message and stopped my "*fabrications.*" I believe that these early episodes of stretching the truth had beneficial effects on me as I grew older.

R32. On a warm sunny day, I noticed something that I had not seen before, something that fell from one of our front yard trees. Someone had apparently stepped on one of them on the sidewalk, and a small amount of liquid came out of it. I tried to duplicate the procedure on another one, and was successful. Then I picked one of them up, and tried to squeeze the liquid out of it as I held it in my hand. This was something that I had never done before and I proudly called my mother to watch me do it again. Well, I got a scolding. Unknown to me, I had picked up and squeezed earthworms!

R33. A wedding party was held in a hall about one city block away from our house. The locals called this hall the "*Sweat Box.*" I did not know what the smiles and gossip were about. Only years later did I realize what I actually witnessed. After the wedding party ended, the bride and groom walked out of the hall. I observed that the young neighbourhood bride, wearing the white gown that denotes virginity, had an obviously distended stomach. I thought at the time it was a large beer belly!

120

R34. One day after our sisters went to school, Nora came over to play. After a few hours I told Nora that I had to go to the bathroom, and Nora innocently followed me in. I threw my "*equipment*" over the toilet seat, and proceeded to relieve myself. I knew that boys were different from girls, and asked Nora to "*show me yours.*" Nora dutifully obeyed my request, and raised her dress well above her knees. I told Nora that I could not see anything, and asked her to raise her dress much higher, which she did. Not knowing what to look for, and not seeing anything to identify, I became annoyed and said angrily, "*You are not showing it to me!*" Nora insisted that she did show it to me. Even though I was annoyed, it wasn't of any great concern, we forgot about it, and left the bathroom to play games.

R35. At Christmas, I was told that Santa Claus would come down the chimney with a bag of toys for me. I looked at a small visible section of the chimney in the living room, and said that the chimney was not big enough to allow Santa's entry. On Christmas Eve, I was shown a piece of Christmas cake and a one-ounce shot glass of whiskey, placed near the base of the Christmas tree. These two gifts, I was told, were for Santa, who would arrive during the night, hungry and thirsty. In the morning, the Christmas cake was gone and the shot glass was empty, so now I thought that Santa really did pay us a visit and leave gifts. What I was suspicious about was how Santa, whom we saw at the Bay, appear at Eaton's within a few minutes' walk—with a slightly different Santa's suit!

R36. One day Metro, my playmate, came over to play. We made a small Native encampment in the living room, with a small tent and a few tiny statues of Natives. The only thing that the Natives needed was a fire to cook with and to keep warm. Metro said that making a fire on the wood floor would not be a good idea. Therefore, I asked my mother if we could make a small fire at the encampment, because it was winter time. It was a good thing that my mother was at home. The poor imaginary Natives had to stay in their camp without heat, but they did have water, although not fire-water.

R37. On a day that Nora came over to play, I needed to have a bowel movement. We proceeded to the bathroom. When I was *"finishing off,"* I told Nora to stand up near the open window, take the used toilet tissues from me, and toss them outside. Nora followed my instructions to the letter—too bad for me. My mother was outside, talking to a neighbour, and saw what was happening. She came in and scolded me. I thought that having these used papers tossed outside for my mother to see was proof-positive that I was toilet trained!

R38. My body movements were always on the slow side. I often heard my mother mention the fact that I was not lightning quick . What lowered my self-esteem in this regard was being compared with an uncle who was slow as well. I was told countless times to hurry up, especially when we were preparing to visit our wealthy Aunt Tina and maternal grandmother in Winnipeg. A tense, rushed feeling is a sensation that I feel to this day. Aunt Tina and her husband, Steve, had two children: daughter Helen and son Orie, short for Orest. This family owned a soft drink plant, six Diamond-T trucks, and a four-door Packard automobile. Their house, it seemed to me, had everything you could ask for: a player piano and many books to read, plus cases of different flavoured soft drinks. I was sharply aware of their wealth and of our comparative poverty.

R39. I heard so much about money, and the lack of it, that I once announced to the family, "*When I grow up I am going to buy a gold fur coat for Mom.*" They smiled. I knew that both gold and furs were expensive and out of reach for anyone in our family at that time.

R40. An adult next-door neighbour, Joe, allowed me to sit on his front steps to talk. Then Joe decided to roll a cigarette for himself and one for me. We lit the cigarettes, and I was very proud of having a whole cigarette instead of a butt, just like an adult. My mother could easily see me from our front door, and while we were smoking, I saw her looking at Joe and me. Knowing that my mother could see me smoking the cigarette increased my self-esteem. I felt more like an adult. My mother could have hollered to stop me from smoking, but she said nothing! I found out in a few minutes why my mother did not try to stop me from smoking. I became so sick to my stomach that I ran home, losing my last meal on the way.

Well, guess what, Stan? That embarrassing event did not stop me from smoking. When the real thing was not available, I would get some store string, wrap newspaper around it, go to the kitchen wood-fired stove side vent, light one end, and then run into the bedroom and hide under the bed for a satisfying, undisturbed smoke.

R41. My sister Vera attended Sunday school at the local hall called the "*Sweat Box.*" Vera obtained permission to take me to this school which was taught by two Catholic nuns. On my first day, one of the nuns came to me and asked in Ukrainian, *"Where would you like to go, to Heaven or Hell?"* I was stuck for the right answer. I knew the two Ukrainian words for Heaven and Hell (Nabo and Paklo), but I was not certain which was which. Knowing that I had to give an answer, I played it safe, and replied in Ukrainian, *"I would like to go to Heaven and Hell."* The nuns and students burst out laughing at my unexpected answer. The nun then said to me, *"You like to travel!"* At that tender age, I didn't know why everyone laughed at my answer, and felt very humiliated.

Stan, who likes to be laughed at? After this single insulting episode, I refused to return to Sunday school at the "Sweat Box."

R42. My mother allowed me to shave my face with a dull knife and soap suds. Shaving made me feel more like an adult. After shaving, I took our triangular mirror outside on sunny days. I reflected the sunlight on different objects, including boxcars, approximately one-half mile away. I wondered why the relatively small mirror cast the reflected sunlight on an area approximately one-quarter the size of the distant boxcar.

Shaving without facial hair was often on my mind. One day our parents bought a frozen half-side of pig. The frozen pig was left propped up against a kitchen wall. I noticed the bristles of hair on the pig's hide, and thought of an idea that might work. I rubbed my cheeks against the pig's bristles in order to transplant the hair growth. I finally obtained facial hair—about 10 years later!

R43. Up until the age of six, I had some happy and unhappy experiences. The impact of some of the upsetting experiences, described previously, caused me to develop a tense, fearful feeling. When I began my first year of public school, there was no kindergarten. I was very frightened. I was afraid of being away from the protection offered by life at home. Fear had, and still has, a debilitating effect on my thinking. During this first school year, I cried so frequently that my crying interfered with my learning. Therefore, I failed the first year of school. My learned fearful behaviour caused another problem, shame. The shame of failing the first year of school lowered my already low self-confidence and low self-esteem. I thought that I was the only one in the class, and also the only one in our family, to be embarrassed by such a humiliating failure at my age!

R44. When I was seven years old, our parents decided to move from the Melrose Street house into their Regent Street side-by-side duplex, one street north. Both houses were almost parallel to each other, and because it was a fairly short distance, I remember carrying lightweight items through a vacant lot to the Regent Street house. The Melrose Street house was later rented. The Regent Street house had larger living quarters and two separate one-car garages. The adjacent 33-foot corner lot, combined with the house lot, totalled a 66-feet frontage.

At the front of this house, on the right side of the veranda, grew a very large horseradish plant. The veranda railing was almost seven feet above the horseradish plant. I would jump from the railing into the horseradish, and was thrilled to hear the air swishing by my ears as I dropped through the seven-foot fall. I was not concerned about damage caused to the horseradish, but my mother was.

She told me, in no uncertain terms, never to jump onto the horseradish again. Thereafter, I would never do the jump when my mother was in sight.

R45. We did not have a Christmas tree for December 25, due to lack of funds. Therefore, my sister Vera and I would check out nearby lanes after Christmas for a tree that had been discarded, drag it home, and set it up for "*Ukrainian Christmas*" on January 7. That is what I called "*living high off the hog, poverty style.*"

R46. During this period I looked to my sister Vera as my protector. Feeling insecure when frightened by someone, I would begin to cry and holler, "*Vera, Vera!*" Nearby children who heard my cries for help mimicked my words to tease me. Their teasing shamed me even more for being so fearful.

R47. With a large back yard area, my parents decided to raise chickens for egg production. Several neighbours became regular customers for freshly laid eggs. My father turned to his beekeeping hobby. Near the fall of the year, we harvested the honey. This was done with the use of an extractor device. Four rectangular honeycombs were placed vertically in this device, and a side crank handle was attached to a horizontal steel shaft. On this shaft, at the centre of the steel drum, was one cone-shaped gear. A second cone-shaped gear was mounted at 90 degrees on a steel shaft. When meshed together they are called mitre gears. When the crank was turned and an adequate speed was reached, you could hear the honey hitting the insides of the drum, forced out by centrifugal force. After the honey was extracted from one side of the four honeycombs, the combs were reversed and the procedure was repeated. When a maximum amount of honey was extracted, it was drained off from a spigot at the bottom of the steel drum into clean containers.

R48. After my two-year stint in grade one, I passed to grade two and ran out of tears. A student named Victor sat behind me. Victor did not seem to know arithmetic very well. Victor who was older and bigger than me threatened to punch me in the nose if I didn't show him the answers to the arithmetic questions and problems. Fearful of being beaten up by Victor after school, I allowed him to see all of my answers.

R49. When I was eight years old, my parents decided to have me baptized. One uncle was a Greek Orthodox priest. The priests of this faith are allowed to marry. His marriage resulted in the birth of two sons and one daughter. For reasons unknown to me, my uncle later decided to become a Catholic priest. After making his application, permission to switch was granted from the Catholic Church officials in Rome. From what I was told, his original parishioners did not take this switch lightly. The pressure on my uncle was so great that to avoid continuing problems, and for safety's sake, he and his family moved to Toronto for some time. Eventually, when the heat subsided, he and his family returned to Winnipeg. Subsequently, for years after his return, he wrote several books. He was also given credit for raising funds to build three Catholic Churches in Manitoba. One of his sons became a Catholic priest and was later promoted to Monsignor.

My baptism took place at our Regent Avenue home. I remember standing on an oak armchair, listening to my uncle go through the ceremony. When the baptism was over, and friendly conversation was near its end, my uncle told my father that there was a fee of 15 dollars to register my additional name.

Well, you guessed it, Stan. My father would not pay, and that name was never registered. Later my uncle returned for visits. He even tried to talk my parents into allowing me to enter the priesthood. My uncle could not persuade my parents to allow me to become a priest.

R50. I did pass grade two in one year, bully for me. Then grade three was the most memorable and satisfactory school year, bar none. The teacher made a big difference to my learning; I was more relaxed. Miss McKellar smiled at me a lot. She showed kindness and was supportive of me and other students in her class. I became quite good in arithmetic and problem solving. Miss McKellar complimented me on some of my drawings. On account of obtaining good grades in arithmetic, Miss McKellar permitted students who had difficulties in arithmetic to sit with me, one at a time, to let me help them out by explaining the methods of multiplying, adding, subtracting, and problem solving. The difference this teacher made in me was astonishing. In a class of approximately 30 students, my report cards usually ranked me in third place. The result of Miss McKellar's beneficial treatment of me was that my brain became more efficient, and I was less fearful. I can only imagine how I might have turned out had Miss McKellar taught me for the balance of my school years.

R51. When we were expecting visitors, and as soon as I heard their car doors slam shut, I would head for a bedroom to be out of sight. The reason was that I knew the visitors were better off financially. The shame of knowing that we were poor by comparison usually drove me into hiding. My dad, having seen me shy away from company before, said to my mother, "*Why does he shy away from visitors?*" Mom never did answer. I wondered why he would not ask me, since I was right there.

R52. It seemed to me that my father saw me as a low-status person, not worthy of being spoken to directly. Perhaps my siblings picked up on our father's attitude towards me. Although, sometimes, Dad would offer me a piece of sandwich, supposedly a gift from "*the bunny rabbit*," after he came home from work. Also, even when I was present, my father would often talk to my mother to have her tell me whatever he wanted me to do. Perhaps he viewed my mother as my slave master, or maybe he didn't have enough respect for me to speak directly to me. This "*second-hand treatment*" by my father made me feel unimportant.

R53. When I was 11 years old, my playmate Eddie took violin lessons. I sometimes went to his house to listen to Eddie practise on his violin. I asked my mom if I could take violin lessons from Leonard D., a music teacher who also taught students at the Bornoff School of Music in Winnipeg. I was happy to get the green light for violin lessons. After a few weeks, at 50 cents per lesson, Leonard D. asked one of his advanced students to listen to my violin playing. Why he had this student listen to me may have been for several reasons, perhaps one was to encourage me. Although Leonard D. talked me into switching the bow from my left to right hand, I wasn't very annoyed, and made fairly good progress. However, a shortage of money slowed down my progress. Each weekly lesson payment was due after the lesson was completed. There were several lessons for which I had to delay payment. Leonard D. never complained about my late payments. For me, not being able to pay for lessons on time was deeply shameful. I must have been doing well learning to play the violin, because Leonard D. promised to get me a music-teaching job at the Bornoff School of Music when I turned 18, provided that I continued with my lessons. A few months after I began my violin lessons, I was diagnosed with acute appendicitis. My appendix was removed by our family physician and surgeon, Dr. Markovitz, at St. Boniface Hospital, in the city of the same name, adjacent to Winnipeg. This hiatus from the violin lessons gave me adequate reason to discontinue the lessons. My strong desire to play the violin was overshadowed by the deep shame of not having the money to pay Leonard on time. My last 50-cent violin lesson from Leonard D. was never paid, a lasting reminder for me of poverty.

R54. Around the age of 13, I wrote to Charles Atlas, the body-building expert, for information on his techniques. When the reply arrived, my mother and sister Vera opened the letter, read the information, and passed it on to me with a smile, which helped to lower my negative self-image even more. I considered the action of my mother and Vera a humiliating invasion of privacy!!!

R55. I was often told by neighbours to put on some weight. In grade 11, I was called *"Skin and Bone"* by a student in the classroom! This comment helped to lower my self-image even more!

R56. Now living at the Regent Avenue home, I had to shop at Figel's corner grocery store. This store, located at Melrose Avenue and Leola Street, was half a city block from home. My mother ordered me to shop at the store quite often, sometimes I made multiple trips in one day, buying one item at a time. Eventually, Mrs. Figel told me to tell my mother to make a shopping list so that both she and I would spend less time on so many single daily purchases. Soon after I mentioned this procedure to my mother, she told me to shop at Verbitsky's corner grocery store, a short distance across the lane. I felt like a well-trained retrieving dog!

R57. About age 15 I found out how to make gunpowder. Four of us had an assembly line to make "*caps*." We used soft copper tubing with one end hammered shut before loading. I measured gunpowder into the open end of the tube, and passed it down the line. Others in the group would very carefully squeeze the open end shut. When night began to fall, we carried our "*caps*" to different street locations in the neighbourhood. In front of a chosen house, we placed one "*cap*" on the cement sidewalk. The "*cap*" was then detonated by our hammering it with the blunt side of an axe. The explosion was very loud, and disturbed the lucky neighbour. Then it was on to the next location, to repeat the process until all our "*caps*" were detonated. We certainly had a "*bang-up time*" with a lot of laughter, at the expense of our frightened neighbours.

R58. Both my parents, separately and on many occasions, impressed upon me their negative views of each other.

When I was home alone with Dad, he would "*anoint me*" with unfavourable comments about what my Mom did "*wrong.*" While my Dad was away from home my mother, usually with my sister Tory, kept up a negative commentary about Dad, for his errors, ill behaviour, and poor financial status. Each parent may have thought, "*I do not say or behave in the nasty negative ways that he or she does.*" For me, these verbal attacks by each spouse on the other left me with less respect for each parent.

R59. For years, after grade 3, I wondered why I could not improve my marks in any of the subjects I studied. At age 15, I felt that "*something was wrong*" with my recall and retention. Therefore, I went to visit our family doctor, Dr. Markovitz, and asked him if he would refer me to a psychotherapist. He asked, "*Do you really think that you need to see a* psychotherapist?" I answered yes. I told him that I could not explain precisely what was wrong with me, and I would like to get this type of professional help. Dr. Markovitz agreed to send me to consult with a psychotherapist. When he told me the hourly rate for the psychotherapist's consultation—$10.00—I had to drop the idea for lack of funds. The evil head of poverty rose up again. Decades later, I was told that my diagnosis was clinical depression. So, because of being poor, I was unable to receive treatment at an earlier age, when it may have been more effective.

R60. A neighbourhood friend Mike, about 10 years my senior, was employed at the Canadian National Railway Stores Department. He suggested that I might be able to obtain employment there. Mike said that my age—16—might prevent me from being hired so he suggested I tell the employer that I was 17. The "*trick*" worked in a way, but the person who hired me had lingering doubts about my correct age. I was employed through July and August and returned to school in early September. Every payday I gave my endorsed cheque to my parents, without asking for pocket money. I turned these cheques over, just as my Mom said she did while living with her parents. Since I had handed in all my endorsed cheques, I asked Mom if I could be rewarded with a pair of skis and ski poles, for the forthcoming winter. The answer was a definite yes! I happily told my friends that I would be getting my own skis.

When winter arrived, I asked my mother for the promised ski equipment.

Guess what, Stan? The answer was a shocking no!!!

My sister Vera standing next to our mother added, "*You are too skinny to ski anyway.*" Daughter and mother looked at each other, each with a sadistic grin. Of course they were "*just kidding,*" but a broken promise at my expense had a devastating effect on my self-esteem. There are some people in our society who claim that the last born in the family gets all the attention and is given everything he or she wants, spoiled, spoiled rotten!!!

R61. Whenever a pimple blossomed on my face, I received a "*compliment.*" My brother Ted would invariably come up very close to me, and with his index finger point to the pimple and say with a grin, "*You've got a pimple right there!*"

Stan, did I feel humiliated? You bet I did!

R62. Our family members usually sought out items that were the best obtainable. If they were too expensive, then cheaper items were "*good enough*" I went along with this attitude. Once in grade school a girl wore a new sweater. Several students gathered around this girl, offering her compliments on her new attire. After hearing the praise given by my schoolmates, I said to the girl, "*That sweater is cheap!*" The poor girl was extremely humiliated! I looked at the faces of the gathered students. They gave me scornful looks. But my comment only reflected what I had heard at home. This episode taught me a good lesson, albeit at the expense of humiliating the girl. The students' scornful looks made me sharply aware of how deeply I had hurt her. So what I learned at home, berating or humiliating someone, was in fact sadistic verbal abuse. This was not the way to gain approval from fellow students! From that incident forward, I tried not to humiliate people.

Stan, it took me many years to break this home learned attitude, and perhaps some still lingers in my brain.

R63. During my early teens, my sister Vera gave me dancing lessons. When our mother happened to glance at us, I usually stopped dancing and walked away from my sister. I would do this in fear of hearing a negative remark from Mom, fear of being shamed for dancing with a woman! My mother never did make a negative remark about dancing with the opposite sex. However, the searing thought of being teased for almost 15 years for having a girl playmate was just as effective as hearing it.

Stan, the shame instilled in me by the "*Nora teasing*" left me with a deep psychological scar!

R64. Marjorie Shapiro, my sister Vera's classmate, became my heroine of sorts. Marjorie, who lived across the street from us, must have received a great deal of teasing from schoolmates because she was of the Jewish religion. I admired Marjorie for getting up and walking to the front of the class, and hollering, "*I know that I'm Jewish* and I'm proud to be Jewish!!!*"

* *Judaism, religious system, doctrine, rites, and customs of the Jews. Funk & Wagnalls Encyclopedia – Volume 14.*

Stan, Marjorie is my heroine! At that age, I often heard disparaging remarks about Ukrainians. However, I did not have the courage to defend myself in any way that paralleled Marjorie's brave defensive attitude.

R65. For the grade 11 graduating ceremonies, everyone was dressed in his or her Sunday best. I had to wear my brother Ted's suit (Ted was serving in the army at that time). The suit did not fit very well, it was obviously too loose for me, another shameful experience for me. Perhaps other people would not feel as embarrassed, but with my background of poverty, I felt like melting into the woodwork.

R66. Soon after graduating from grade 11, I dressed up and began my ecstatic quest for half-decent employment. I applied to the National Employment Service, located in Winnipeg and was interviewed by a man who quizzed me thoroughly. I may have told him that my mother wanted to channel me into university. It is true that obtaining an advanced education is a very worthwhile and noble endeavour. It was also true that we lived in poverty, and the thought foremost in my mind was, overwhelmingly, to become financially independent. No doubt then, after saving adequate money, I would have enjoyed attending university. The interviewer ordered me to go back to school! Upon hearing these words, I became more depressed because I had failed to obtain employment. Then, under protest, my mother actually took me in tow to United College in Winnipeg. I felt like a slave being forced to enrol and my mother paid for the tuition. I felt that I was the only student who had a parent enrolling me, Shamed Again. I told my mother many times beforehand, there is something wrong with me and I know that I will not make it. She sounded somewhat annoyed when she asked, *"How do you know?"* I felt like a horse being led to water who would not drink.

R67. I was brainwashed by my mother's desire for me to study medicine. I felt like a programmed robot, encased in a transparent cage, following a channelled pattern of life, dictated by my well-meaning mother. After I entered grade 12, at times I felt as though I were in an almost dreamlike state of mind, stunned. Once in this stunned state of consciousness, I walked into the path of an oncoming car. Luckily, the driver was in a much better state of mind than I was. He slammed on the brakes, the tires squealed, and the car stopped inches away from my legs.

Studying medicine is very expensive. I asked my mother, *"Where will the money for books and tuition fees come from?"* Her answer was, *"Never mind!!!"* If there were adequate funds for my education, where were they, and why couldn't I be told that they really did exist? Was this blind, unrealistic hope?

Remember, Stan, I could not get a mere 50 cents every time I took a violin lesson!

Perhaps I was our mother's hope that I would be the only one in the family to obtain a higher education, a laudable goal. However, the choice was not mine, and this idea was an almost impossible quest for me with my emotionally fractured mind. Sometime later, my Dad, sounding annoyed, asked me, *"How long are you going to go to school?"* My answer was, *"As long as I have to."*

R68. My Dad, just prior to my Mom's *"Back to School Order,"* was, I thought, more realistic. He wanted to sell the Melrose Street house, and buy Bagley's house which was about one-half mile east of our Regent Street home. This vacant house had adequate land surrounding it. Dad wanted to start a chicken ranch at that location and I was delighted with the idea. My father saw my enthusiasm for the chicken ranch concept, and he gave me a broad, agreeable smile. This type of business was a way to make some money. However, Mom decided against selling the Melrose Street property. Once again we were stuck in poverty.

R69. One day, Mom and Dad agreed on one thing, when I was about 18 years old. It was time for me to get married! My reply took less than a nanosecond. I said, *"I have seen how your marriage has turned out, and I don't want to follow with a repeat performance."* Years later, I told my older brother Joe about my rapid response to our parents' revolting marriage suggestion. He agreed emphatically, with one word, *"Good!"* Joe must have had good reason to agree.

Stan, there are at least three reasons why I took a dim view of getting married at age 18:

1. I was laughed at by Nora's mother and by my mother for having a female playmate.

2. The trauma of being teased and laughed at, merely from hearing the name "*Nora,*" for almost 15 years from my mother and older sister Tory, left a feeling of deep shame in me. Years later, my psychotherapist told me, that being laughed at is one of the worst insults that a person can receive!

3. The years of experience of being raised in a family whose parents were verbally abusive to each other and to me, could hardly be seen as a model conducive to a happy marriage. As the years passed, my resistance to marriage, very slowly, turned to a more positive view. My opinion was changed as I observed many happy marriages in our society.

R70. After completing grade 12 at United College in Winnipeg, I took the pre-medical course at the University of Manitoba. Naturally, being in my "*fogged*" state of mind, I could not acquire marks high enough to qualify for medical school. Failure to enter medical school increased my sense of shame, and lowered my self-image. Yet I remained tethered to my mother's desire for me to study something "*medical.*" I felt "*strapped in a mental straitjacket!*"

R71. Still doubting the ability of my "*stunned*" mind, I was determined to see a psychotherapist in order to get a professional opinion of my mental capacity. This psychotherapist was friendly, knowledgeable, and, almost a chain smoker. After a few appointments, he sent me to a pleasant lady who put me through several oral and written tests. After completing the tests, I left the building to go home and found myself lost. I listened for noise from vehicle traffic and walked in that direction. Reaching the heavy traffic area I was at a main thoroughfare, Portage Avenue. I was no longer lost and headed for home. I met with the psychotherapist again after he received the results of my mental tests. The psychotherapist used an analogy to indicate my test results. He said that, "*I was running on 10 cylinders out of a possible 12.*" Therefore, I believed that "*my brain was two bricks short of a full load.*"

R72. At the age of 21, I decided to go to Vancouver to study bacteriology at UBC. My brothers Joe and Ted were living in Vancouver and, with some financial assistance from my parents, helped pay for my tuition and other expenses.

R73. I thought it was normal to contact and live with my brothers. Unknown to me at the time though, I was not welcome. I was not aware of their unspoken negative attitude towards me, because nothing was said directly to me in this regard. Many years later my sister Vera said to me, "*You and I are treated like members of a different family*". I agreed.

Stan, I always felt like the lowest one on the totem pole or not even on it.

R74. When my brothers and I had a discussion, my point of view was usually opposed. Their opposing views of my opinions on various topics became so frequent that I decided to test them over periods of time.

For example, months after offering my opinion X, when their opinion was Y, I purposely took their former Y position. When I supported their original Y position, which they formerly claimed was correct they now said that the Y point of view was wrong!   Therefore, I told them to call me by my new name Wrongo, which obviously described their opinion of me. Whenever they disagreed with my viewpoint, I answered, "*Wrongo strikes again!*" It was unlikely that my viewpoint was always correct, but it seemed that only their opinions were faultless, and even interchangeable. They usually supported each other's viewpoint.

R75. A real estate agent named Bill suggested that "*In order to make some money for your education, you should borrow $5,000 from your brothers. With this money, you could run a hotel rental business which I have listed for sale.*" When I asked my brothers for the loan, their answer was no! Some years later, when our nephew asked to borrow $50,000 from my brothers, the answer was *yes!*

R76. Once, while some friends were visiting us, one complimented me. Joe replied in an annoyed tone of voice, "*He is not so smart.*"

R77. At age 22, I thought that it was mandatory to learn how to dance in order to meet a girlfriend. I went to a popular dance studio owned by a pleasant pair of instructors. During one of my last dance lessons, the instructor said to me, "*Someone must have been very mean to you.*" I was surprised to hear this observation. Initially, I thought that the instructor's statement was invalid. At a much later date, I learned that well-experienced dance instructors can observe, sense, and feel excessive tension in their students. My overly tensed body muscles did not allow for smooth dance movements. Years later, I mentioned this dance instructor's statement to a psychotherapist. The psychotherapist, without hesitation, said, *"Yes, they can feel the tension in one's body."*

R78. When alone with mutual friends of my brothers, someone asked me, *"Why do your brothers talk about you that way?"* My answer to this question was always the same: *"I don't know."* I never asked what the negative comments were. One closer friend, Adam, referring to my brothers' negative comments about me, said, *"They want to put you down, suppress you!"*

R79. Jack, a friend who lived in the same rooming house as we did, told me that my brothers Joe and Ted complained to him about my choice of words when I spoke. My brothers never complained to me about my working vocabulary. Jack told me later that he explained to my brothers that the learned words I used were a normal consequence, or influence, of a higher education.

R80. When going for a walk with Joe and Ted, I noticed that, if ever a pregnant woman were in sight, her condition provoked words of derision and laughter from us. Now, years later, I look at this attitude as a deviation from normal attitudes towards procreation. This distorted view of pregnancy had a negative effect on our behaviour, and not one of we three brothers had children. Personally, I felt that if I impregnated a woman, I would feel so shamed that I would change my name and move to a different location. My distorted attitude towards procreation was caused by almost 15 years of sadistic teasing for having a GIRL as one of several playmates in my early childhood. However, this sadistic teasing did not stop me from being attracted to women. Of course, I understand that none of us would be here if it weren't for sexuality and pregnancy. The preservation of the human race is dependent on sexual attraction between men and women, with the potential for creating children.

It is also true that, with all biological organisms, there is some kind of fertilization process causing the development of offspring or new life. Human life is like an ever-expanding river of people, with some passing on and new life being brought forth to the planet. This most natural and wonderful process is one in which I took no part, for the painful reasons stated above.

Stan, the sadistic teasing mentioned above distorted my procreation instinct.

R81. I was at the University of BC, about to enter my fourth year of Arts, majoring in bacteriology. After a few weeks of this first term, I knew that I did not have adequate funds to continue. Therefore, I recovered my first term dues and obtained employment at the Murray Plywood Mill, where I had worked previously. My plan was to work at the plywood mill for one year, save some money, and return to UBC to complete my degree. After I had gone back to work at the plywood plant for a short time, my brothers Joe and Ted made a very attractive offer to me. They had purchased a Cardero Street rooming house business while working in Vancouver as bus drivers. The Cardero Street house required an interior "*facelift.*"

Joe and Ted suggested that I quit my work at the plywood plant and do the painting wallpapering etc., in the rooming house, while they continued in their jobs. I also did some grocery shopping and cooked suppers. By agreeing to their terms, I would be entitled to one third of the net profit. My brother Ted added, "*You will make enough money to go back to university and even buy a car.*" This certainly sounded like an extremely fair deal to me, and I agreed to their terms, a very enticing verbal agreement.

With my refunded university dues, my brothers and I bought paint, wallpaper, and supplies for the rooming house renovation.

In time, the Cardero Street house renovations were completed, and the rooming house business was sold for double the purchase price. Life was looking good. The profit was used to purchase property at 1648 Davie Street, the current location of London Drugs.

Now, get this, Stan. My brothers decided to have this property placed in my name only!

Their reason was that I did not have a record of being gainful employed; therefore, when this property was sold, I nor they, would not have to pay capital gains tax. Not knowing any better, I trusted my brothers and went along with this agreement. Work progressed on upgrading the interior of the house, and the exterior was painted by a friend with a pressure sprayer. Not long after the renovations were completed, the house was put up for sale—in my name only and when sold the money would be paid to me!

When a buyer came along to purchase the house, which was still only in my name, I was told by my brothers that now I had to sign an owner's release form. The Vancouver Land Titles Office keeps records of such transfers. The release form I signed transferred the property back to my two brothers, and only then was the property sold.

After the sale of this house, on a sunny day in front of the property, the three of us had a conversation. Joe said to me, "*We cannot pay you any money from the sale of this property, because we need all of it for the purchase of the house on Alberni Street.*" Not being paid wages, I began to wonder when I would be paid the verbally agreed amount of one third of the net profit.

Stan, not long after moving into the Alberni Street house, Joe said to me, "You are not getting any money from the sale of these properties." I replied, "I thought you would say something like that."

So there I was, Stan. Not only had I quit my plywood plant job, the original verbal promise of one third of the profit was broken, so going back to university and "even buying a car" were impossible. What did I get? Board, room, cruel deceit, a broken verbal agreement!!!

Guess what, Stan? I obtained work as a security guard at Oakalla Prison Farm for three years. Later, I found work in the home renovation business. I worked in Vancouver, Calgary, and Regina, where I met my wife, Cecile.

R82. When the Alberni Street property was sold, there was enough money to place a down payment on a three-storey apartment building at 1547 Comox Street. When my brothers were in the process of moving from the Alberni Street house to the Comox Street apartment block Joe said to me, "*There is no room for you in the apartment block.*"

R83. I moved from the Alberni Street house into a light housekeeping room. After my brothers moved into the apartment block, Ted approached me with a new deal. He said to me, "*We will let you rent a one-bedroom apartment suite for the same price you are currently paying for the light housekeeping room.*" I accepted this generous offer, and moved in.

Much later, I found out why I was given this "*generous rent offer.*" There were so many vacancies in the apartment block that every available dollar was required to meet the mortgage payments.

Stan, surprise, surprise! Now there was space for me in the apartment block!!!

R84. After the sale of the Comox Street apartment block, my brothers purchased the Surf Apartment Hotel located on Beach Avenue, next door to the Sylvia Hotel. I was now married to Cecile. I was hired to work at "*the Surf*" at an original wage offer of $550.00 per month, mainly to renovate kitchen cabinets and replace bedroom carpeting. Ted wanted to keep his bus driving job for several years until he was old enough to retire from it. Later, Joe talked Ted into quitting his job against his will. SURPRISE, for some reason my wages dropped to $200.00 per month. The purchaser of the Comox Street apartment block hired me to manage their building.

R85. I discovered that, at least 30 years earlier, my brothers had called me by two "*pet names.*" I learned this while talking on the phone to a Comox Street tenant named Paul, who used one of these names just before he hung up his telephone as he spoke to someone with him. Initially, these names were used only between my brothers and their friends. Later, my brothers greeted me with a grin and one of these names almost every morning when I arrived to work at the Surf. Their friends were kind enough to call me by these names in whispered tones, just loud enough for me to hear. The pet names were "*Booby*" and "*Asshole.*"

R86. During "*the Surf period*" a real estate salesman named Rod became close friends with us. When the time was ripe, Rod was determined to sell the Surf and spent a good deal of money advertising the business. Rod became such a close friend that my brothers promised to reimburse him for all his Surf advertising expenses, even if someone else found the buyer. As it turned out, a friend who was not in the real estate business found the buyer. I was present when Rod visited to collect the money for his advertising expenses, as promised verbally by Joe and Ted.

Guess what, Stan? My brothers decided not to pay Rod for his advertising expenses. Well, Stan, Rod was not the type to settle for a broken promise. In a threatening tone of voice, he said, "In a court of law, a verbal promise is just as valid as a written promise!" After hearing this statement, without any argument, a cheque was made out payable to Rod for the total amount of his advertising expenses. As Rod left with his cheque in hand, he said, "I will never do business with you two again."

R87. Social drinking of alcohol in our society, in general, is considered quite acceptable. It is seldom compared to taking drugs, and I often wonder why.

Stan, during "the Surf period," I began drinking heavily. I usually drank with my two brothers, Joe and Ted, and their friends. Nobody forced me to drink!

I became less inhibited when I drank. I felt more relaxed, and in time I looked forward to drinking. I didn't realize that I was becoming addicted to alcohol. I even felt that there was something wrong with people who did not drink at parties. My reasoning was that so many people whom I knew drank, and that those in the minority who did not drink were missing out on "*the fun.*"

Stan, my on-again-off-again heavy drinking lasted approximately 5 years. Prior to this, I drank only on Saturday nights and did not get "loaded."

Approximately 30 years ago, I stopped drinking, almost "*cold turkey.*" Today I understand that because of my depressed, fearful, shamed state of mind, drinking alcohol was the wrong solution. The correct, or proper, solution came, and is still coming, from "*The Gem Quality*" psychotherapists.

R88. Prior to the sale of the Surf, Ted told me that when this business was sold, "*We will give you something.*" Soon after the sale of the Surf Joe came over to make their offer to Cecile and me. The offer was a new television set, and the choice of the model was left to my wife Cecile. The TV set she chose cost $800.00! After Cecile made her TV choice, Joe and Ted had a conference regarding the gift, and their decision was, "*It is too expensive.*" Their next offer was that Joe would buy a new TV for himself, and we would be given his used TV. I countered with, "*Keep your TV for yourself.*"

The Surf building and property was sold in about 1968, for exactly $500,000. The original asking price was $495,000. The buyer, with me present, asked Joe to toss a coin for $5,000. Joe won the toss, so the price went to $500,000, and the net profit was approximately $250,000.

Our friend Aziz, who found the buyer for the Surf, said to me, "*If you were not given $800 by your own brothers to buy a TV, I will not even get a bottle of Scotch for a finder's fee!*"

Stan, Aziz was dead right. Once, during a conversation with his brother Budruh, Aziz, referring to me and my brothers, said to Budruh, "He is smarter than both of them." Perhaps, but the truth was, at that time, I was too trusting of my two brothers.

R89. Ernie, a lawyer and a mutual friend, had a talk with me in his automobile.   Ernie was sympathetic as we discussed my brothers' broken verbal promises.

R90. During an evening walk, I mentioned to Cecile, "*It is not right to cheat a brother, and I think I should consult a lawyer regarding Joe's and Ted's broken promise of net profit sharing.*" Cecile's reply was, "*It is not right to take legal action against family members.*" I guess she was correct from her point of view. If I had taken legal action, as Rod alluded to doing, I would then have had my two brothers and Cecile in opposition. However, had I taken legal action, Cecile and I would have benefited financially.

R91. After the Surf was sold, I left the Comox Street apartment managing job. Cecile and I moved to our present location and I found employment as gardener at the Pacific National Exhibition. On my two days off from that job, I worked as a security guard. My compelling reason for having two jobs was to save enough money to purchase a house requiring renovations, which I was capable of doing.

After saving adequate funds to purchase a house, I checked the listings of houses for sale in the Vancouver Sun. I phoned one owner about his property, asking for the sale price, which was approximately $29,000. I said that I would call back to arrange an appointment to view the house with Cecile. I asked Cecile when she would have time to look at this property, and did not receive an answer, which puzzled me.

Much later, I learned that many people, including myself, feel very insecure for different reasons. One way in which people gain a sense of security is by saving money in a bank. Seeing their bank account gradually increase gives these people a sense of security. Other methods—for example, investing money in property—are deemed by some as too risky. And everyone is entitled to his or her own opinion.

So, under the circumstances mentioned above, I felt compelled, without any reply from Cecile, to drop the idea of buying a house to renovate, a speculative concept with some chance of financial loss, but also a possibility of monetary gain.

R92. One day, on a bus, I met Fred who was a stock salesman. I was skeptical about investing in highly speculative stocks, and against my better judgment I purchased some penny stock that Fred recommended. After purchasing the stock and feeling very worried, I phoned Fred every day. Unfortunately the stock rose in price, I sold it at a profit, and I became "*hooked.*" As time went by, I bought and sold stocks with some gains—and many losses.

R93. While still employed at the PNE, I decided to volunteer with St. Paul's Hospital Auxiliary. I was assigned to spend time with patients on Tuesday evenings after work. Some of the patients had few visitors and so sought more companionship. One lady wanted to play cards with me every Tuesday evening. Those patients without visitors could watch television, if they liked the programming, while others sat alone, perhaps dwelling on their illnesses.

I soon realized that I was attending to only one patient, the lady who liked to play cards. After a few weeks I asked the head of St. Paul's Hospital, Auxiliary, Ella S., for permission to obtain entertainers to perform for the patients.

I thought of phoning seniors' residences, and found that some did have entertainment programs. I visited some of these seniors' homes, and was offered some names and telephone numbers. Through them, I obtained the names of others who were willing to offer their skills, from solo musicians, Italian, Scottish, and Ukrainian dancers, and choirs, to a variety of bands.

For a little over nine years, I overcame the "*one volunteer to one patient problem.*" I've been told by some SPH employees, that the patients greatly appreciated the entertainment, which was a refreshing break during their recovery in the hospital.

R94. After working at the PNE for approximately 17 years, I slipped on a hillside while carrying a hedge trimmer and suffered a left shoulder rotator cuff injury which required surgery. The surgeon thought that I might not regain the use of my left arm. However, with excellent physiotherapy at SPH, I recovered, although not enough to return to work. Therefore, I had to retire just short of retirement age.

R95. Now, having a great deal of spare time, I tried to think of something worthwhile to do. I noticed that some areas of the Lower Mainland had neighbourhood police offices, but there were none in Vancouver's West End. I wrote letters to 19 cities with neighbourhood police offices, asking how effective their operations were. The letter replies were all supportive of their neighbourhood police offices. Therefore, I asked some friends to volunteer part-time to obtain local residents' signatures for our petition for a police office in our neighbourhood. Later, we had a meeting with the Vancouver City Police, and one inspector broke the news that there would not be a neighbourhood police office in the West End for at least ten years. I visited the New Westminster Police Chief and the RCMP in North Vancouver–their opinions of neighbourhood police offices were both positive. After approximately one year, the first neighbourhood police office was established in the West End Community Centre on Denman Street.

R96. Soon after purchasing a VCR at Eaton's, I heard of a new VCR feature, with a feature called commercial advance. The advantage of the CA is that 80-90 percent of recorded commercials are played through at such a rapid rate that the main programming is interrupted for only several seconds. Of course, I returned my newly purchased VCR to Eaton's and received a $550.00 credit.

After waiting for over a month to buy the VCR model with CA, I went back to Eaton's to pick up the desired set. The salesman with whom I had dealt was on sick leave. I spoke to another salesman and their manager, who both told me that they had NO record of my $550.00 VCR credit. Eventually, after I hired a detective to trace the ill salesman, the Eaton's staff contacted their ailing salesman, and he admitted that he did give me the $550.00 credit!

My brother Ted was aware of my VCR credit problem, and I decided to phone him regarding the VCR credit news.

Without talking about the VCR credit, Ted said to me referring to our one bedroom apartment, *"You know, you've only got one room there, and the only place you can read is in the can"*—i.e., the bathroom.

Stan, for me, this was a very painful insult, which I consider sadistic verbal abuse!

After hearing this comment, and still in a state of shock, I cut the conversation short. Then I phoned my brother Joe and his wife, who also lived in a one-bedroom suite. I quoted Ted's comment about our suite, and Joe said to me, *"Ted says some mean things"*!

R97. Years ago, I had an intestinal polyp removed through my abdominal wall, at UBC Hospital. One day during my hospital recovery, five people came to visit me: my wife, Cecile, my brother Ted and his wife, Avis, and two friends named Joe and Larry. We talked for some time in a visitors' room. A hospital staff member came by and called me by name. As I stood up and walked a few steps, Ted said aloud for all to hear, *"Gee, you've got skinny legs."* The visitors were numbed into silence.

Ted, and others like him, rely on acid remarks as a way of increasing their self-esteem. People who use such tactics become caught in their vicious cycle of verbal aggression. It makes for uneasiness, and distances the victims, with the possible result of loss of friends.

R98. We invited my brother Ted and his wife, Avis, to our place for a Sunday dinner. All went well for some time. Ted began to complain about two friends, Johnny and Katie, who had given some money to their son Kenny to help him out with his plumbing course. Ted and his wife were against helping out anyone in a financial way. Ted's continued comments against Johnny and Katie were so extended that I said, "*Let them do what they want.*" Knowing that it was not Ted's money being given to Kenny, it was entirely Kenny's parents' decision to do what they wished with their money.

Later in the evening, Ted stood in front of where I was seated and said to me, "*We have a lovely home and a car.*" I believe that this was said to insult me for not being supportive of his opinion that Johnny and Katie should not have helped their son financially.

R99. *Stan, after we successfully established the community police office in the West End, I came across information about a new type of equipment for firefighters. In order to proceed with fundraising for this equipment, I had a charitable foundation incorporated in Ottawa, in 1996, called Human Horizons.*

The equipment allows a firefighter to enter smoke-filled rooms to find anyone overcome by smoke and fumes. Fire Chief T., felt that the Fire Department could make use of five such units. Captain W. had contacts who could help us raise the necessary funds. Five of these units would have cost approximately US$250,000.

Soon after, I was informed that Chief T. had just retired. I telephoned the new Fire Chief about the acquisition of the required equipment. His response was, *"That equipment is too high tech."* So we had to drop the idea of fundraising for this equipment, despite its life-saving potential.

Another type of equipment I found out about was a new type of breast cancer detector. The claim was that a physician could use this equipment in his office, and determine if a patient had breast cancer within 20 minutes. I turned this information over to a doctor who, at the time, was the head of a cancer agency. I did not receive a reply from him.

Stan, the next type of equipment I came across was called a Ventricular Assist Device system (VADs). It is used on certain cardiac patients. Knowing that you have a heart condition, I think you will find this device important. Therefore, I'll give you more details on it than on the two items mentioned above.

- The VAD system is a temporary artificial heart, or blood pump.
- It helps the damaged heart to increase and maintain normal blood circulation for the patient.
- With this pump providing normal blood circulation, the cardiac patient's vital organs can function at their best capacity before, during, and after corrective surgery.
- Because the pump maintains normal blood flow, the cardiac patient's chance of survival is greatly increased.
- The blood pump is best used in cardiac surgery for the following conditions:
    a. Cardiogenic shock

b. Myocarditis

c. Cardiomyopathy

d. Acute myocardial infarction (resistant to less effective therapy)

e. Pretransplantation

f. Acute heart transplantation rejection

R100. Stan, my mind just jogged me back to grade nine when I purposely chose to study French instead of Latin. The reason being, I knew that Latin was a prerequisite for studying medicine which was not my choice.

When my mother realized that I was not taking Latin, "a fix" was arranged. My sister Vera told the Latin teacher that I MUST study Latin. During class the teacher called out aloud to me, that I must start talking Latin, embarrassing you bet!!!

Chapter 13 - How I am
Recovering from Shame

Most of the following information taken from a psychotherapist.

S tan, for many years I blamed family members, and significant others in my past, for breaking their promises, and for ridiculing, shaming, and frightening me.

I was, as I wrote earlier, *"in the loop"*; that is, repeatedly *"talking in circles"* by blaming family members for what they actually did to me. I felt justified in blaming these people who used, and still use, verbal forms of mental abuse on me. Their painful, negative comments were often in my mind, and I was trapped in a crippling resentment response to them. I was *"trapped in the loop,"* thinking about past painful experiences, over and over again, without trying to develop solutions to these problems!

I know that I must let go of all these past and some current resentments. My self-damaging thoughts are as painful and corrosive as acid being poured on my festering emotional wounds. Also, these resentments can inflict psychosomatic illnesses on me.

For me, merely saying *"I forgive you"* is an inadequate method of freeing myself from the painful effects of verbal abuse perpetrated on me.

My techniques for *"forgiving"* verbally abusive people:

- As I learn more about the causes responsible for my own fear and shame-based behaviour, I am able to understand and acknowledge that these verbally abusive persons in my life have themselves, for similar or different reasons, been emotionally crippled as a result of their early childhood conditioning.

- I am coming to realize that because of their learned behaviour, these "*significant others*" are doing the best they can, just as our parents did. And as I slowly learn, and understand, more about why people behave the way they do, my resentment, fears, shame, and guilt diminish at a directly proportional rate.

A. Recovering From Shame

Stan, one way for me to handle my shame is for me to develop my sense of self-esteem, so that what other people think of me does not matter so much anymore. What does matter is what I think of myself; that is, my self-definition or self-concept.

Other people can be critical and judgmental of me in an effort to make their own viewpoint(s) look like reality. These viewpoints are sometimes based on their own perceptions of reality, which may or may not be true. Such viewpoints are based on their own perceptions of reality.

The Judeo-Christian-Muslim ethic is to "*love your neighbours as yourself.*"

Fortunately, Stan, many people do practise this ethic. They have attitudes of compassion and understanding towards other people.

In that environment, shame is minimal because we feel that other people love us and accept us, and are not judgmental, just as we love and accept them, and so they are not judgmental in return.

Shame tends to arise in environments where people are not following the dictum of compassion.

The Buddhist central idea is compassion. Amongst Buddhists there is little emphasis on shame as an emotion. There is a lot of emphasis in Buddhism, as in Christianity, to develop one's own sense of self, and to develop compassion for other people.

So, Stan, I can let my mind dwell on these ideas. And as I evolve in terms of the foundations of my own self-esteem, my shame diminishes. And also, if I choose friends and acquaintances who are ethical and compassionate, shame is less likely to arise.

A lot of my earlier experiences, of course, are derived from my family's dynamics, but now I can discriminate and choose not to spend time with people who are negative and judgmental, thus making my feelings of shame less likely. I have a choice, I have control and the ability to be in the driver's seat of my life. I can diminish my fear and shame by increasing my self-esteem. I have my own sense of who I am choosing to keep company with. That is, people who are more compassionate and loving.

These ideas will lead me to reflection and thoughtfulness, and I can move forward beyond shame!!! I can take some time to just really relax, to let my conscious and unconscious minds help me overcome this challenge!

Shame is said to be a learned emotion that often begins at a very early age. It is most detrimental when it comes from those who are closest to us: parents + siblings + significant others.

*S*tan, *as the youngest of five children, I was very impressionable, and shaming during this period has had long-lasting effects on my behaviour which are difficult, but possible to overcome! As a child I was deeply shamed, and carried my painful beliefs as though they were cemented into the inner world of my brain, where they remained into my adulthood.*

Common shaming phrases used to control a child's behaviour:

- Shame on you!
- Why can't you be like Jimmy?
- You are a hopeless child!
- You are a sissy!
- You are acting like a baby!
- You are a selfish brat!
- You are a cry baby!
- You are a hateful little boy!
- You are spoilt!
- You are a naughty brat!
- You are just trying to get attention!
- You are a whiner!
- You are a little terror!

As a child, my self-concept was formed mainly by what family members said about me. My behaviour was treated as second rate, and eventually I grew up feeling inferior and unimportant. As a shamed child, I avoided socializing and expressing many of my emotions, because I did not feel *"good enough"* about myself. Extreme shame caused me to become emotionally depressed and anxious.

This repeated shaming to control my behaviour caused me to dwell on my inability to please. And so, I became very obedient to please others in order to gain some degree of approval and affection.

When I was shamed for being "*bad*" nobody explained their feelings at the time, and I had no way of relating to my parents' or older siblings' emotions. Without any explanations of their irritable "*feelings*" regarding my "*bad behaviour*" I had difficulty in relating to and developing empathy for other people's feelings. When family members shamed me, I learned to avoid shaming by becoming submissive to adult demands. However, if our parents had had adequate respect for each other—and for their children—we siblings would have likely developed a more caring attitude towards other people.

At a very early age, as a baby, I tried to have my basic needs met in the only ways I knew how to communicate my emotions: by crying, anger, sadness, etc. Perhaps if my parents had been able to understand these early behaviours for what they were, they might have been less tempted to shame me. With less shaming, parents could devote more time to teach their children greater happiness and self-confidence. A child likes to mimic the behaviour of adults, so if our parents had been able to vocalize their feelings without shame, we siblings would likely have imitated our parents. And, as a consequence, our parents would have received reciprocal emotional benefits.

Shamed children who years later become parents often perpetuate their learned shaming experiences by passing them onto their children. So this new generation of parents, endowed with the humiliation of shame inflicted on them by their parents, is likely to perpetuate the cycle by shaming their own children. However, if these parents could recall the painful humiliation of being shamed as children, their memories might help them avoid the damaging effects of inflicting shame on their own children.

Raising children is a very demanding task made much more difficult by the absence of previous experience. It is quite normal that parents' anger will erupt from time to time. Parents have the option of taking out their anger on their children with shaming or trying to channel it off by talking over their problems with their spouse, or with appropriately qualified counsellors/psychotherapists.

With some exceptions, children who are raised in dysfunctional families will later, as parents, tend to raise their children in ways similar to the inadequate ways they have learned from their own parents.

Sadism

Sadism is defined as emotional gratification gained by inflicted physical pain or humiliation on someone. It may also be defined as finding enjoyment in being cruel to someone. Some people are friendly without being abrasive. Other people, who at times are genuinely friendly to others, become verbal abusers of their chosen victims by using open or subtle humiliation.

Victims like me have suffered from such humiliating talk are left with psychological scars that can last for a lifetime. Depending on the amount of verbal abuse, it tends to lower the recipient's self-esteem, causing him or her to become confused, or uncertain about him- or herself, and about the self's true abilities.

The verbal abuser either denies the hurtful remarks, or claims that they were of little or no consequence. For example, when a family member used verbal abuse on me, it was often combined with a grin, and followed with an explanation that, "*I was only kidding!*" This meant that it was I who was at fault by feeling hurt by their comment; "they" were innocent of hurting me even though they had inflicted the verbal abuse!!!

*H*ow do you like that for rationalization, Stan? I recognized verbal abuse used on me and on other members of my family. Well, Stan, under these circumstances, would you be surprised to learn that I started to use verbal abuse myself? Verbal abuse is designed to make the scapegoat feel submissive, worthless, and powerless. You will read, further on, that the verbal abuse hurled at me had a "branding iron effect," leaving lasting emotional scars such as fear, shame, and low self-esteem.

Stan what I experienced during my formative years was fear, shame, verbal abuse, and an inadequate loving atmosphere. Under such conditions, these feelings, as well as forgotten ones, are stored in a part of the brain called the amygdala. These deeply ingrained sensitive feelings can easily be triggered by less severe related stimuli, often causing a person to overreact. However, we can be trained, over time, to obtain more control over the amygdala, to react less severely to more realistic threatening situations. That is, the left frontal lobe can, with conscious effort, gradually retrain or "tame" the amygdala.

Here is one example of "taming" my amygdala, by going into a hypnotic state given by a psychotherapist. Stan, read the following very slowly, calmly, and warmly, in the way it was spoken to me.

Psychotherapist:

So imagine, Bud, you are sitting on a park bench during a beautiful day in June, and let your mind wander, and wonder about yourself as a kid. Then you see a little guy coming up the path, and as he gets closer, you recognize him as the *"younger you."* And he is happy, yet with a little sadness, a little fear, and you ask him to sit beside you. Then you put your arm around him, and he snuggles up to you and you say to him, *"I'll take care of you, I will make things safe and secure. And you can let go of the pain, the hurt, the shame, and fear, and in their place will be love and faith, and hope, and trust."*

In a way, we all have to raise ourselves in the end, in one way or another, we have to hold ourselves close and it's a wonderful picture, something to see yourself as a young kid, and you give yourself a big hug!!!

Your adult self can help your *"kid-self,"* and the wounds can heal, really heal, so the kid's pain disappears as mist when the sun comes out, and you feel whole and carefree and happy!!! And you both begin giggling and laughing, telling stories to each other. You have a great old conversation about all kinds of things. And it's an amazing process that your relationship to yourself can alter your own experience, such that you begin to get curious, adventurous, and you want to learn everything there is to learn about, living life fully and joyously with energy, a sense of exploring things, really confident and secure. A presence that other people can feel aware, you just feel whole and happy and wise, in ways of your own relationship with yourself!!!

Now you can relax, deeply and profoundly, Bud, and you can view those images in your own way, such that it touches your heart and changes the pathways in your mind, and so you can heal yourself in many ways!!!

It is sad when abusers resort to degrading people to prop up their own self-esteem. When we understand their motive, we know that verbal abusers are in some kind of pain that makes them behave in that hurtful manner so that their pain is being redirected at their victims!!!

Once you understand the reasons behind verbal or other abuses, and have suffered from them, you can move on to becoming your own best friend and literally elevate your self-concept because you missed out on some fundamental love. And the way you can make up for that is to be gentle and compassionate with yourself, with all your shortcomings, and giving yourself unconditional love!!!

It is a strange idea, but we all have a relationship with ourselves. It seems puzzling on the surface, but it is true! And abusers who humiliate other people to increase their self-enhancement, don't understand that really, self-esteem is an inside job. It is not going outside and making themselves better by standing on other people's shoulders or sadistically humiliating other people. That is not a lasting way to build up one's self-esteem!!!

The German dictator Adolf Hitler, an abuser, used Jews, homosexuals, gypsies, mental patients etc., as scapegoats to make the German people feel superior. This calculated strategy of racial, physical, mental-fanatic superiority was used because, in any movement, a *"crusade"* moves along quicker if there is a targeted group to hate. This calculated strategy was based on the false premise of the superiority of the Aryan race. The irony of this concept is that the members of the Aryan race are blond and blue-eyed, and Hitler, along with many of his henchmen, was NOT blond or blue-eyed!!!

One of the easiest ways for an abuser to feel superior to their victims is to humiliate them! Convenient targets are those who are younger, weaker, or smaller in size, or people of a different race, with something about them that is *"different"* or *"unusual"* or *"vulnerable"*—for example, not looking much like others in a family in skin colour, facial features, etc.

Stan, verbal abuse is found in some television shows such as "All in the Family." Archie Bunker, the head of this family, put down:

- his wife, Edith, calling her "*Dingbat*";
- his son-in-law, Michael, calling him "*Meathead*"; and
- his daughter, Gloria, for marrying Michael.

The TV audiences really laughed at the misfortunes of the show's characters. This indicates how easily we can slip into laughing at the pain of other people by insulating ourselves from their obviously hurt feelings. However, how well are we insulated when others laugh at our personal adversities?

A few examples of verbal abuse used in our family:

- When my sister Vera began to wear eyeglasses, she overheard our mother and sister Tory agreeing that "*Vera looks ugly wearing glasses.*" To this day, Vera takes off her eyeglasses just before answering a knock on the door.
- Once our father came up to my sister Tory and called her "*Grey Eyes.*" I could see from Tory's face that she was hurt. I said to her, "*When I grow up to about 20 years old, I'm going to beat up Dad.*" The irony is that Dad had the same colour eyes as Tory: "*Grey Eyes!*"
- Our mother once said to my brother Joe, "*If you do not do what I say, you will have to leave home.*" The frightening prospect of being "*kicked out*" of his family prompted Joe to run away to the home of our maternal grandparents who lived many miles away.

As I build my own self-esteem, I know in my heart that I've done good things for other people. Giving to people, without expecting anything in return, is a beautiful act of love, which enhances my self-esteem!!!

Self-esteem is built from love, faith, hope, imagination, creativity, and the ability to wonder about things. The Buddhists say that our job is to evolve and become wise. And while we are doing it, we should stay light, bouncy, and humorous; in other words, we shouldn't take ourselves too seriously. Every day is a chance to grow, learn, and discover—all of which can create the pillars of a person's self-esteem and compassion for others.

B. Improving My Attitude

The information below is taken from conversations with a psychotherapist.

This is a list that I read periodically, in an attempt to improve my behaviour and attitudes:

Stan, during an appointment with a psychotherapist, I wrote the following instructions. In order for his words to have a greater impact on us, I "personified" them to read as though You and I are now following his instructions.

- When I am able to admit my undesirable behaviour, I dismiss it and try to change for the better in the present, which is the only time to make changes.

- When the opportunity presents itself, I try to be kind and helpful to people, and I sometimes get the same courtesy in return. That is the golden rule: *"Do unto others as you would have others do unto you."*

- I offer genuine praise, without exaggeration, to those people who exhibit positive attitudes and worthwhile accomplishments.

- I avoid ridicule of people as much as possible. As I learn more about my own behaviour, I also increase my understanding of others.

- When an opposing thought is presented by someone, and I decide to offer an opinion, I try to use a calm voice and usually begin with, "*From my experience, I have found that ...*" Using this approach is a much less confrontational and more acceptable way of presenting my interpretation or opinions.

- Although still a bit limited when I am depressed, my ability to laugh and be more upbeat attracts more people to me by helping to put them into a happier frame of mind.

- I am trying to smile more, and to add humour when appropriate. By being more optimistic, I tend to make myself a more pleasant companion.

- When I am definitely wrong, I try to admit that I am. By doing so, I am seen as being more credible, and I therefore often gain more respect from others.

- I try to limit my opinions to comments on what is "*right*" about a person, rather than what is "*wrong*" with that person.

- As I try, and as I slowly become genuinely more understanding and accepting, I receive the equivalent from like-minded people.

- At times when I have unintentionally harmed someone, I have found that the "*wrong*" often returns to me.

- When others have seen that I have let go of trying to control them, it allows them to make their own decisions, and they then become responsible for the consequences of their own actions and decisions.

- I, like many people, have a need to belong to someone, or to a group of people. Even in our family, every member learned that when the anger and arguments subsided, we were all still functioning members of our dysfunctional family!

- Very slowly, as I let go of my shame, fear, anger and resentments, my energy level increases and is available in the "*present.*" This relatively new change has pushed ajar the heavy door of the dark, depressing past. This allows in some fresh air and bright light to stimulate my mind in the "*present moment*"!!!

- I am also learning how to forgive myself for indiscretions and acts of poor judgment in the recent or distant past.

- I am trying to develop a worthy opinion of my "*self.*" When I give compliments without exaggeration, to people deserving them, I feel more appreciated and accepted just for being myself.

- Generally, as these needs are satisfied, I find that life has more meaning, and I begin to feel more competent and useful. This enables me to make better choices in directing my life.

Dr.G. a Psychotherapist

Of eight psychotherapists, seventh, the amiable Dr. G. after three years of therapy asked me if I had noticed much improvement in myself. I replied, "*To tell you the truth, I do not see much improvement.*" Dr. G.'s reply was, "*Here is NO HOPE.*"

And so with this psychotherapist's negative opinion of me, I was convinced that I was a hopeless case. I never went back to see Dr. G. because I was completely assured that seeking help from him or any other psychotherapist was hopeless.

Much later my family physician Dr. C., recognizing my depressive state, and after much prodding, eventually convinced me to see a certain psychotherapist having a reputation for being very competent. Little did I know that I would soon hit the proverbial "*Jackpot*" by seeing Dr R.

I have had many successful appointments with this psychotherapist. I believe that Dr. C. and perhaps divine intervention guided me to the gem-quality psychotherapist.

This psychotherapist is a man with very high ethical and professional standards. Once when I complained to him that I wasn't improving a great deal he did not answer with "*Here is no hope.*" Instead he replied, "*Perhaps you are not completely aware of your current condition.*"

This psychotherapist seems to radiate a penetrating inspiration in me. Also, with his progressive therapy, I believe that he is a veritable modern day oracle.

During some of my appointments Stan, I wrote out important explanations relevant to my upbringing and other topics which may be of value to you.

In short, after receiving therapy from several psychotherapists, without exaggeration, it was only he who substantially reduced my long standing fears and deep depressive state.

C. Solving My Conflicts

From THE psychotherapist:

Our accumulation of life experiences, knowledge, and culture which influences our current thoughts, opinions, and interpretations is called *"our frame of reference."* Each person's frame of reference is unique, and this is why my point of view may be similar to, but not necessarily in complete agreement with, that of another person. Therefore, when attempting to solve conflicts, I find it advantageous to take into account the fact that frames of reference differ. This is another example of *"personalizing"* his words of wisdom i.e. inserting the word *"I"*.

If I do not seek to develop solutions to my conflicts or problems, I will remain *"in the loop."* Being in the loop is the state of repeatedly voicing my problems without seeking any solutions!

- If I deny that a conflict exists, I will not be able to resolve the problem!
- Conflicts can be settled by brainstorming. Accepting the ideas of others involved gives these significant others the opportunity to participate with equality!!!
- I try to go through the pros and cons of the ideas without allowing anyone to be authoritarian! I evaluate each idea from both children and adults. I am careful what I say *"Yes"* to!
- I take action. I make a plan to see that the idea works, and make changes, with all the participants included.
- I try to admit orally what is *"right"* about a person, rather than limit my opinion to what is *"wrong"* with their current or past errors and behaviour!
- I forgive myself, as well as others, for negative attitudes, sadistic verbal abuses, and misdeeds of the past!

Step 1. The first thing I do when solving an interpersonal disagreement, or conflict, is discover where the other person is coming from—which requires a lot of listening!

- Basically, I try to crawl into that person's head, universe, and way of thinking, and I let him or her realize that I want to understand him or her. To do this, I reshape, or review, or restate where I think he or she is coming from!!!

- Then I ask him or her if I have the correct ideas about his or her position, and if not, I ask if he or she could possibly correct my thoughts about his or her opinions.

Step 2. Then I can ask them if they would like to know what I think, and would they be able to listen long enough for me to explain my viewpoint, so that I can explain where I am coming from.

- Then I can say, after my explanation, "*Can we somehow make a 'win-win situation' out of this?*"

Step 3. Sometimes it has to be done as a series of steps. I ask the person to think it over and then we will get back together later.

- Often this is the artful way of doing it because I am not telling them anything negative, simply to "*think it over.*" And they do think it over if they are sincere!!!

- They often come back to me, and their position will have moved a little bit from what it was. And hopefully, in the meantime, my position will have moved a little bit closer to their position.

- So I start getting the idea, and the exciting idea is that I can move closer and maybe when we combine our positions or ideas, an overall more comprehensive idea will begin to take shape, and we can combine our separate realities into some larger reality.

- So often, reality is seen in a narrow way, whereas it should be seen in a broad, detailed, or comprehensive way.

- Sometimes things appear one way, and they end up another. Sometimes I can say things to people and they think, "*Who are you to say that to me?*"

Step 4. Conflict resolution really does not work unless I have rapport, or a sympathetic understanding with people, and trusting people is part of that rapport. My rapport is necessary so that I can build up a relationship of trust!

Step 5. Another thing that helps conflict is humour, the idea that somehow there is an interesting and yet funny aspect of the conflict. When I joke a little bit and get the other person to laugh with me, it takes a lot of "*heat*" out of the situation.

Step 6. Now, creativity is something that comes when I ask questions. I can say to the person, "*You know, I've done a lot of thinking about this subject and my question for myself, and perhaps for you, is how to find a 'win-win situation' when your position is X and my position is Y.*" It is possible to develop a 'win-win situation' so that at the end of the day our combined realities will end up creating realities in a more comprehensive way?

Step 7. It is well known, that in every situation there is a little bit of "*black,*" and a little bit of "*white,*" and a hell of a lot of "*grey.*" And when I recognize that this is the case, I think about:

- Listening

- Asking questions
- Brainstorming
- Trust
- Humour
- Creativity

S tan, these are some of the elements that are useful in solving conflicts!

D. Improving My Mood

The information below is taken from conversations with the above mentioned psychotherapist.

S tan, this is one of many important topics that I remember from my psychotherapy sessions. I thought it may be of interest to you.

Endorphins are one of a group of chemical compounds that occur naturally in our brains. They have pain-relieving properties similar to those of opiates. After adequate exercise, I experience *"a higher mood"* caused by an increased level of endorphins.

Another thing that *"kicks off"* the endorphins is laughter, wit, and comedy. That's a wonderful way to change my internal environment: increasing endorphins with more laughter, comedy movies, etc.

Another way of increasing my endorphins is just by remembering good things that happened to me, things that I am proud of!!!

Yet another way to increase my endorphins is to watch a beautiful sunrise or a spectacular sunset, or simply to notice the fragrance of pine trees and nature's beauty, which is refreshing.

One of the neatest ways to keep my mind occupied is to present it with new things. I look forward to each day to open my mind to things such as:

- Languages
- Crossword puzzles
- Sudoku
- Different cultures
- News about political events, to *"keep my finger on the pulse"* of what is going on in the world!!!

I enjoy things like reading novels and non-fiction too.

I enjoy journeying inside myself and deciding such issues as self-esteem and what it is based on a non-judgemental approach to myself. I can be firm with myself, and yet not really judgemental!

I can support myself and be my own best friend. I can visualize the kind of future I want, and it is important to stay in the precious present and to have goals that pull me along!

Another way to improve my mood is by slowly developing amnesia or forgetting my painful experiences, whether they occurred in the present or the past!!!

To develop and reinforce this happier mood, I recall and write down, in short form, old and new successful experiences, whether great or small, and enjoy the good feelings they bring!!!

And in order to maintain this improving frame of mind, I keep this list and read the positive reminders especially when I feel somewhat "*down.*" Then, as I begin to feel more "*upbeat,*" I sometimes think of another happy experience, and write it down to build up my happy experience list!!!

A nd, Stan, this effort to achieve a happier outlook or mood by writing down happy experiences is possible at any age, provided that you read what you write. Reason: the human brain has an innate capacity for change, and positive mood change makes for happier thoughts!!!

The happiest cultures in the world are those that have a philosophy of staying, or living, in the present moment!!! More traditional cultures, like those of India and parts of Europe, tend to focus a bit more on the past.

North American cultures often focus on the future, and people worry themselves silly about what will happen next day, next week, next month, next year:

- And what am I going to do when I retire? That is when I am really going to live!
- And I'll start to be happy when I do X, and when is X not accomplished I can keep on dreaming up new X's which I really don't intend to fulfill.
- When I get enough money I won't have to worry about it.
- When I get this health matter looked after I will be happy!

1. Laughter

S tan, the information below is taken from conversations with the above psychotherapist:

We've often heard that laughter, and even the anticipation of laughter, has beneficial effects on our minds and bodies. It is often said that *"laughter is the best medicine."* So why don't we laugh more? Perhaps some of the following information will help us develop, or enhance, our attitude to laughter.

Our sense of humour changes as we mature physically and mentally, and increases with our knowledge and experiences. What we experience as humour is usually restricted to what we know about our culture and community, and the individuals who are part of it.

Stan, did you know that humans are not the only ones who laugh? Now it is said that lower animals, such as chimpanzees and rats, are capable of their own form of laughter, which is also related to their brain's "reward system."

What Happens When We Laugh?

When we laugh, 15 facial muscles contract, and muscles in the upper lip are stimulated. Our respiratory system's irregular intake of air can make us gasp. When laughter is strong enough, it can activate our tear ducts. A rare negative experience of extreme laughter is involuntary incontinence.

Laughter's Psychological Benefits

Laughter can have a temporary, cathartic effect on unexpressed emotions such as fear, anger, and sadness, which are not on one's mind during periods of mirth or hilarity. Such negative emotions, when not expressed, can cause biochemical changes that can have a harmful effect on our bodies. Laughter is an easy way to shake off annoying thoughts and replace them with inner peace, making you feel livelier, healthier, and more creative.

Therefore:

- Try to be friendly with people who have a good sense of humour.

- Spend more time watching funny movies or TV, or read jokes that make you laugh.

- Try to increase your own sense of humour, but not at someone else's expense. Using verbal abuse and sarcasm against anyone to generate laughter becomes an implement or tool to vilify, malign, or give the victim a "*verbal black eye*." Usually the perpetrator is the only person who enjoys this type of laughter.

Did you know?

- When in company, laughter brings about greater harmony.

- Laughter lessens any hostility by encouraging more friendly behaviour.

- Laughter is often contagious; we usually laugh because someone else is laughing, and therefore more bonding occurs in a group.

- Women tend to laugh more during speeches if the speaker is a man.

- We laugh more when we are with people than when we are alone. So we can conclude that laughter in company improves interpersonal relationships.

Laughter's Physiological Benefits

- Muscles, as they contract in the thoracic wall, abdominal wall, back, respiratory system, diaphragm, and legs, get an excellent workout with laughter. These muscle contractions, in turn, elevate the flow of oxygen into the blood, helping the body to heal.

- Laughter helps clear the respiratory tract of mucus and increases immunoglobulin A in saliva, which helps to protect bacteria from entering deep into the respiratory tract.

- Laughter reduces blood pressure, and vascular blood flow is increased.

- Laughter assists in balancing all immune system components, which ward off diseases.

- Laughter has the capacity to lower certain stress hormones that suppress the immune system.

- Blood platelet production is lowered by adequate laughter. These platelets can cause arterial blockage, and so raise blood pressure, so we want to lower them if possible.

- Laughter increases T-cells. T-cells destroy bacterial and viral infections, and destroy tumors;
  - o the protein gamma interferon, another disease fighter;
  - o the production of B-cells, which create disease-destroying antibodies; and
  - o the secretion of our growth hormone.

- Laughter creates and releases endorphins, our body's natural painkiller. Endorphins also give us a sense of well-being, also felt after exercising. This sensation is similar to the effect of opiates.

- Laughter lowers our secretion levels of cortisol. Cortisol, a hormone increased by stress, suppresses our immune system and has a negative effect on memory recall.

The Power of Laughter

S tan, the following is the classic story of how Dr. Norman Cousins saved his own life with the abundant use of laughter.

Norman Cousins is known to say that laughter is like "inner jogging."

Norman Cousins wrote a book called "Anatomy of An Illness." It is the story of his laughing himself well. He speculated that laughter was a potent healing force. He and his doctor worked together and looked at various tests like the SED rate, which is a general measure of inflammation, because he had a severe type of arthritis: acute ankylosing spondylitis, which is a degenerative, inflammatory, spinal disease.

The SED rate is the measure of how well they were doing with their treatment plan, which included watching comical movies, Groucho Marx, Candid Camera, etc. The SED rate, or erythrocyte (red blood cell) sedimentation rate (ESR), is a test to screen blood for diseases. It is done as follows:

- A blood anticoagulant is mixed into a sample of a patient's blood.
- This mix will now not allow the blood to clump up, or coagulate, thus permitting the blood cells to freely settle down because of the pull of gravity. This blood mix is then poured into a special glass tube, marked in millimetres.
- The blood mix is then allowed to settle for one hour.
- The SED rate, or ESR, is the speed at which red blood cells fall to the bottom of the glass tube.

One comedy seen by Dr. Cousins involved a delivery man who took a package to a resident who was sitting in his rocking-chair on an empty lot, reading a newspaper. The only other thing on the lot was an upright door frame, with a door in it. When the delivery man arrived, he looked at the resident on the empty lot, rocking and reading his newspaper. He rang the doorbell and the resident got out of his rocking chair, came to the door, signed for the package, thanked the delivery man very much, and went back to his rocking chair with his newspaper and the package. The delivery man stood outside the door in total shock.

Later, Norman Cousins measured his SED rate and changes in his cortisol level, which, as time went on, became a little lower because high cortisol is stress-related. His cortisol level went back to normal!!!

Cousins was able to monitor certain parameters, like the SED rate, the cortisol level, the white blood count, level of pain, his sleep, and other variables. They all changed for the better—because of increased laughter! For example, Cousins discovered that only 10 minutes of belly laughter while watching the comedian Groucho Marx gave him an extra two hours of pain-free sleep! And two hours of belly laughter while watching Candid Camera gave him an anesthetic effect resulting in pain-free sleep!

The main purpose of these laughter experiments was to find out if laughter alone, without the use of pain medication, could diminish pain. As you may have gathered, it worked well!

Norman Cousins wrote several articles on the power of laughter. Then he started writing on the power of other beneficial emotions and characteristics like hope, faith, love, compassion, curiosity, and creativity. He began to list the positive emotions, and was able to search in the literature and find other evidence that these helped to improve the human immune system, the body's defence system, as well as other aspects of health. He wrote an abridged version of his book which appeared in the New England Journal of Medicine, the most prestigious medical journal in the world.

Dr. Cousins became an honorary graduate of medicine at UCLA in recognition of his valuable work on the role stress plays in pain, and how de-stressing your self can help you in surprising ways.

Any kind of activity that increases your endorphin levels is also good for pain control. When you start feeling good about yourself having fun and laughing, your body benefits greatly. Think of funny events in your life that will make you laugh.

Condensed Benefits of Laughter

Stan, there is a link between brain cells and the immune system's cells. Laughter reduces stress hormones. Stress hormones suppress our immune system!

- Laughter allows us to "*break loose*" in a positive way. This "*breaking loose*" helps to vent our stress and frustrations, making us "*feel better*"!
- Laughter decreases physical tension!
- Laughter increases both neurotransmitters and the painkiller endorphins!
- Laughter increases leucocytes (white blood cells), which destroy our body's invaders!

2. Laughter Experiences

"Take a Message!"

*S*tan, three of my wife's relatives from Regina came to spend their holidays in Vancouver and on Vancouver Island. While in Vancouver, my wife and I took these relatives out for supper at the top of the Landmark's Revolving Restaurant. The tower offers a spectacular view. On our way to this restaurant, my wife told me in no uncertain terms, "Make certain that you pay the supper bill!" I got the message.

Upon arrival at the restaurant, I took the hostess aside and asked her, *"Would it be possible for you to notice when our company is almost finished dinner, then come to our table and pretend that there is a telephone call for me? And instead of going to the telephone to answer the non-existent telephone call, I will leave our table, and follow you to the cash register and pay the total dinner bill."* The hostess smiled, and agreed to this strategy.

Later, at the appropriate time, the hostess walked up to our table and said, "Mr. *Bozyk, there is a telephone call for you!"* This was our agreed strategy for me to leave our table and pay the bill. A second after the hostess announced that there was a telephone call for me, I replied, *"Take a message!"* The hostess laughed so hard at my unexpected reply that she actually bent over at the waist! While the hostess was bursting with laughter, my wife said to me in an authoritarian tone of voice, *"She is not your secretary!"* This statement only served to escalate, reinforce, and amplify the hostess's laughter.

Well, what more could I do? I left our table and followed the laughing hostess to the cash register, paid the bill, and gave her a well-deserved tip for her *"Oscar-Winning Laughing Performance."*

"In the End"

I once attended a Dale Carnegie course and gave this speech:

One day I came home from work with a severe lower back pain. I lay down for half an hour to relieve the pain, but it did not subside. Then I asked my wife to get the bottle of 'HEET' liniment to rub on my belt-level back area. Thanks to my good wife's tender application of the 'HEET' liniment, the pain began to subside. About 30 minutes later, not feeling the excruciating pain, I took a shower.

After a few minutes in the shower, I washed my lower back where the 'HEET' liniment had been applied. The soap and water loosened the 'HEET' liniment. While in this standing position, it seemed that every applied drop of 'HEET' liniment was channelled between my rear lower cheeks, and entered the orifice on which I normally sit. The burning pain was indescribable. I felt like running in order to escape the pain, but that act may have resulted in a fine for streaking!!!

Then I thought of drying off the burning tender area with a towel. The towel was *too* rough and intensified the pain. Then I thought of drying off the *"tender burning spot"* with cool air from an electric fan. I plugged the fan's cord into the wall outlet, crouched down, and *carefully* backed towards the fan.

*S*tan, *visualize this. I had to move backwards with caution to avoid fan blade contact with my "vital parts." Otherwise,* contact with the rotating fan blades would mangle and lacerate, turning me into an instant soprano!!! Women assuming this crouch would be in a safe position, not having hazardous appendages.

Lucky for me, the fanned air did the trick, and without the loss of a single 'jewel'!!! The extreme burning pain diminished, and soon after, I had no pain in that area. Some people still think that childbirth is painful. If they had 'HEET' in the seat, they would really know what pain is!!!

So, friends, if you ever use 'HEET', or any liniment for back pain, always keep a fan on hand!!!

Happiness and Laughter Quotations

- "A well-guarded mind brings happiness. Those who are free from all worldly desires will attain Nirvana. Never covet what others have. It is a deadly sin which grows away from all happiness. Learn to be happy with what you have." Buddha.

- "The first step in seeking happiness is learning. We first have to learn how negative emotions and behaviours are harmful to us and how positive emotions are helpful. We must also realize that these negative emotions are not only very bad and harmful to one personally, but also harmful to society and the future of the whole world." The Dalai Lama.

- "It involves an inner discipline, a gradual process of rooting out destructive mental states and replacing them with positive, constructive states of mind, such as kindness, tolerance and forgiveness." The Dalai Lama.

- "The person who knows how to laugh at himself, will never cease to be amused." Shirley McLean, actress/dancer.

- *"What soap is to the body, laughter is to the soul."* Yiddish proverb.
- *"Laughter is a tranquilizer with no side effects."* Arnold H. Glasgou.
- *"One loses many laughs by not laughing at oneself."* Sarah Jeanette Duncan.
- *"Against the assault of laughter nothing can stand."* Mark Twain, humorist, lecturer, writer.
- *"Laughter is an instant vacation."* Author unknown.
- *"Happiness is the meaning and the purpose of life, the whole aim and end of human existence."* Aristotle.
- *"Stan, to be happier, if you ever take a laxative and a sleeping pill at night, you will be much happier if you put on running shoes before going to bed!!!"* Bud, your friend.
- *"Our prime purpose in this life is to help others. And if you can't help them, at least don't hurt them."* The Dalai Lama.
- *"All traditions of major religions basically carry the same message that is love, compassion, and forgiveness. The important thing is these should be part of our daily lives."* The Dalai Lama.
- *"Good humour is one of the preservatives of our peace and tranquility."* Thomas Jefferson, third US president.
- *"If you keep thinking of all the ways in which others cheated you, fought with you, degraded you, or angered you, your heart will forever be full of hatred. Learn to let go, and be happy."* The Tao of Happiness.
- *"Happiness is the meaning and the purpose of life, the whole aim and end of human existence."* Aristotle.
- *"Humour is mankind's greatest blessing."* Mark Twain, humorist, lecturer, writer.

- *"One of the basics of human nature is that we are a social animal. So our life is based on community. So good relations with others, good companions and life, social kind, therefore (this) brings happiness."* The Dalai Lama.

Stan, the Dali Lama believes that a person becomes happier by practising compassion, caring, forgiveness, kindness, and tolerance.

E. Improving My Memory

The information below is taken from conversations with a psychotherapist.

Stan, about 20 years ago it was discovered that we do not have a complete store of neurons (nerve cells) during childhood. Our brain, and other organs, maintain a supply of stem cells that can generate new neurons through a process called neurogenesis (neuro = nerves + genesis = creation, creation = the development and growth of nerve cells). It was found that neurogenesis goes on throughout life in all regions of our bodies, including our brains.

Stem cells are not specialized cells. However, they can change into specialized cells when properly treated and required for any part of the body—for example, blood cells, brain cells, etc.

Progenitor cells are found in post-natal cells. They can, through several cell divisions, produce distinct cell images. They share some features with stem cells, but their self-renewal is limited compared with the unlimited self-renewal of stem cells.

Oligodendrocytes' main purpose is to cover nerve fibres (axons) to protect the central nervous system, which transmits information throughout our bodies.

Neurons, or nerve cells, are specialized cells that have dendrites, a cell body, and axons. There are billions of them in every body's nervous system. Impulses of information are created mostly by chemical plus some electrical processes. These chains of information are brought into the cell body by dendrites, and sent through the neuron's cell body. The information is taken away from the cell body along the axon to its terminal and sent across the "*synapse gap*."

Billions of the brain's neurons do not touch each other. Neurons communicate their messages by secreting neurotransmitters, which are made by a neuron's cell body. These nerve impulses of information travel to and from all parts of the body. In response to a signal, neurotransmitters can cross the synapse. They are recognized and selected by the appropriate receptors on cells' surfaces found on neurons, muscle fibres, glands, etc. Neurotransmitters perform all the main functions of life except reproduction. Neuron secretion of neurotransmitter messages or impulses is what we sense as feelings, learning, memory, thoughts, emotion, and other functions of our brain. The combination of the brain and spinal cord is called the central nervous system (CNS).

Memory, Stan, is the brain's complex process of recalling experiences or information that you have learned. It's the body's storage depot.

Memory can be divided into two categories:

1. *Short-term memory.* This stores information for seconds or minutes. Short-term memory is purposely fragile otherwise our brain would become loaded with useless information such as TV ads. It is meant to keep an average of seven items. This is why you can often remember a new telephone number, but only for a few minutes.

2. *Long-term memory* involves the conscious or unconscious effort to retain information. The long-term memory is personally meaningful to you and you make an effort to retain it. It also requires a conscious effort to recall stored information—for example, skills that you have used so often that little or no conscious effort is required when you have to use them.

S tan, four areas of the brain are very important in forming and retaining memory:

1. The hippocampus, one of the brain's most primitive parts, is involved in complex physical aspects of behaviour controlled by emotions. It plays the largest role by processing information as memory.

2. The cerebral cortex is the brain's outer layer. Long-term memory is stored in different areas of the cerebral cortex depending on the type of information being processed—for example, problem-solving, language.

3. Amygdala. There are two. They are roughly almond shaped and are located in each cerebral hemisphere. The amygdalae look after processing our emotions, such as mood, instinct, and feelings. They are connected to the hypothalamus which controls body temperature, thirst, hunger, water balance, and sexual function. The hypothalamus is also closely connected with emotional activity and sleep.

4. The frontal lobes consist of the motor cortex which controls voluntary movement. Further to the front are the prefrontal lobes which are responsible (especially the left lobe) for learning, behaviour, personality, and judgement.

Memory involves communication throughout the brain's network of neurons (brain cells). Neurons are specialized cells that can transmit chemical/electrical nerve impulses (of information) from one location in the body to another. There are millions of neurons in our body, all activated by neurotransmitters.

Maintaining Memory

In order to recall your stored memory information, the brain must reactivate the same pattern of neurons that were used in storing it. The more often you try to recall this specific information, the easier it becomes to fetch or retrieve it.

In order to store new information into your memory, you must concentrate intensely.

Researchers were impressed with a group of nuns, all in their 70s, 80s, and 90s, because they had very little Alzheimer's disease compared with the incidence among the general population. *Very few nuns* who did crossword puzzles, played Scrabble or bridge, and generally kept their minds active developed Alzheimer's disease.

Such pursuits as exercise, novelty, humour, learning a new language, and challenging our minds to remember things helps to increase neurogenesis—and also reduces high cortisol to bring it back down to normal levels. Cortisol impairs the functioning of the hippocampus by decreasing the number of cells there. Novelty and exercise coax the stem cells into developing new neurons in the presence of other cells in the hippocampus. These new duplicated neurons (or brain cells) serve the same original short-term memory purpose. Neurologists now think that the hippocampus downloads, or transfers, memory information while we are sleeping and dreaming. And one of the functions of dreaming, they think, is to transfer the short-term memory from the hippocampus to the cerebral cortex where it is stored forever as long-term memory.

So, the more your hippocampus remembers, the more the cortex remembers.

I try to keep noticing different things, tuning into details, being alert. I notice the buildings I walk by every day that I didn't notice before, the flowers that I didn't notice before and the flashes of colour at sunrise and sunset. By doing so, my mind stays alert and registers these things, and the hippocampus then works on them and sends them up to the long-term memory department in the cerebral cortex. Then they are there to be retrieved when I attempt to recall them.

So, anything I can do—turn on the French TV station and listen until I can begin to understand some of it; deliberately look up words that I don't know the meaning of and finding out their meaning; learning part of a language, even without becoming proficient in it—that brings a memory-enhancing benefit. I can play Scrabble and cards, sometimes where strategies are required to remember what cards are down and what cards my opponent has in his hand. And just by believing in myself, believing in my memory, it is amazing what I can do.

And remember, any form of exercise increases endorphins, those chemicals that make you feel good naturally. And when I start feeling good about myself, I can feel good about all kinds of other things, too. And I will understand that having fun, and laughing are very, very valuable activities! I can think of funny events in my life to make me laugh, events that touched my heart with pleasure and joy and laughter.

I've heard it is possible that genetic inheritance may also play a role in our behaviours. The best current information on genes, and their relationship to depression, is that bipolar disorder has a strong genetic origin. For other kinds of depression, the jury is still out. No one has found a single gene responsible for depression or anxiety or alcoholism or personality traits of various kinds. The latest thinking is that it is not as simple as one gene, it is probably an array of genes that turn on and off!

Now there is a *"gene chip micro-array technology."* This process allows researchers to record the interaction of up to thousands of genes at the same time while they subject a person to, say stress, and then look at the response of 15 or 30 genes to see if they all respond differently to stress. And the responses, of, say, the 30 genes with the proteins they secrete or manufacture, which is what genes do, show patterns. There is more interest in large patterns of gene response from 15, 30, 40, or 50 genes. Geneticists can then look at certain patterns of genetic response. Things as complicated as depression and anxiety, or introversion and extraversion probably arise from an array response of very many genes. How much is nurture and how much is nature is very controversial. Geneticists look for genetic causes, while psychologists highlight learned belief systems of the family and significant others.

We often hear that each person is unique, and this certainly appears to be so. Past personal experience leads me to believe that my current behaviour is the result of a combination of biology, psychology, family birth order, financial status, environment, and cultural factors.

Everyone experiences different amounts of stress, depending on circumstances. However, prolonged elevated levels of emotional stress increase the secretion of the stress hormones cortisol, prolactin, and ACTH, and this causes memory decline in the hippocampus.

Dr. Robert M. Sapolski, a neuro-endocrinologist at Stanford University, proved that high levels of cortisol damage and kill some of the cells in the hippocampus during the day.

Stan, with physical exercise, novelty, learning a new language, and mental gymnastics, we can actually create new cells in our brains. In other words, by doing so, we can cause a positive effect on our genes!!!

Anything that makes us think we are not so flexible is incorrect. The newest information tells us that at any given time we are the masters of our destiny more than we ever thought possible! At one time, it was thought that we were born with our assignment of neurons, and that was it; they just died off as we aged. But now, not so! We can create new neurons probably not only in the hippocampus (memory, learning, etc.), but in the cortex, too (thinking, action, etc.). When we do that, we can change our belief system, our moods, our memory, just by doing things like:

- Exercising!
- Being kind and loving to ourselves!
- Learning new things!
- Being curious!
- Laughing a lot!

So, Stan, we have reason to be encouraged that we have the ability to grow, develop, and evolve, and to be light and happy, curious and creative. Most recent findings are sources of strong optimism for people affected by depression.

The short-term memory, for example, remembers a conversation from a few minutes ago, or the phone number that was just learned, or a name or something that was learned by reading a magazine article. These memories are initially held in the hippocampus, and eventually, often at night during sleep, the hippocampus transfers the memories to various areas of the cortex for long-term memory.

As mentioned above, though, prolonged elevated levels of emotional stress increase the secretion of cortisol, prolactin, and ACTH, which causes damage to the hippocampus cells. Low stress and medium stress don't damage the cells in the hippocampus. I can remember concepts that I learned a few days ago, or many moments ago, and they come to me easily and effortlessly. And that means that my hippocampus is functioning in an optimal way. Therefore, because I want to increase my memory, I am *decreasing* my tendency to rush!!!

I have to confess, though, that from time to time my mind goes blank, usually when I am thinking of something or other, but on a different topic. I can go blank, for example, when I am having a conversation with somebody. What has happened during that *"blank"* memory moment is that something in the conversation drew me to some memory in the past, or a worry, or an idea that's not exactly fitting into the present context. So when I try to remember where I was, it's often like trying to remember a dream upon awakening in the morning.

I am probably not *"blank"* in the sense that there is nothing going on. What's probably happening is that I am drifting off like a student does during a boring lecture. Something in the lecture, perhaps, made the student think of being on a beach somewhere. And then, when he tries to remember the current lecture content, it only seems as though his mind went *"blank."*

The state of mind is an interesting thing. Some people go in for a written exam and go *"blank."* It's their anxiety that takes them into an anxious state of mind. In their anxiety, that anxious state of mind, they can't access their calm state of mind. So they get trapped in the anxious state of mind and they can't get out of it easily. And in the anxious state of mind, they don't have recall of the things that they have in their normal state of mind.

S*tan, for many years I have experienced moments of my memory going "blank."*

There is an idea called *"state-specific learning"* or *"state-dependent learning."* The research is interesting: for example, they can teach people nonsense syllables to the point where they remember 90% of them while they are intoxicated. And when they are sobered up, they can remember only 50%. But if they get them drunk again, they remember about 90%!!!

So, states of mind don't necessarily communicate with one another. It's almost like the information to be retrieved is in the wrong file drawer. When I am anxious or drunk, or just drifting off somewhere, I just can't remember where I was—a blank state of mind!

In short, the degree to which I can lower my stress level, and slow down my urge to rush, is directly proportionate to my memory capacity.

F. Lowering My Stress Level (part one)

The information below is taken from conversations with a psychotherapist.

S*tan, rushing steals our peace.*

History

The fight or flight response experienced by ancient humans worked well because those people had to fight their enemies and/or flee from predatory animals for their self-preservation. Unfortunately, it also puts stress on both mind and body.

The earliest scientific studies on stress were conducted by Hans Selye and Walter Cannon, who used animals exposed to "*stressors*" such as temperature, surgery, and restraint. Dr. Selye was born in Austria in 1907. In 1932 he moved to Canada and became a staff member at

McGill University in Montreal. Later, he became the director of the Institute of Medicine at McGill.

In 1936 Selye, by then a world-renowned endocrinologist, began researching what he later called *"stress"* at McGill. Together with a team of assistants using thousands of experimental animals, Selye had mice injected with a variety of irritating organ extracts. The extracts caused:

- swelling of the kidneys' adrenal cortex,
- stomach ulcers, and
- shrunken thymus glands at the base of the neck.

Dr. Selye observed that humans with different diseases showed symptoms similar to those found in the injected experimental test mice. Selye used the term *"stress"* to describe how the traumas of the mice, injected with irritating organ extracts, reacted on the adrenal glands, stomach, and thymus glands. The organs affected became overactive, causing disruption of the body's homeostasis, or body equilibrium.

Dr. Selye claimed that a stimulus is a *"stressor"* if it results in a *"stress response"* in the recipient. He identified two types of *"stress"*:

1. Positive stress, or *eustress*, is a pleasant, mirthful laughing state that produces healthy, positive emotions. It can enhance performance and achievement, and enhances well-being. Eustress in managers makes them show greater competence in leadership which leads to greater staff cooperation.

2. Negative stress, or *distress*, can be the result of a bullying atmosphere, where threats, coercion, and fear may be the result of inadequate management skills. In the workplace, this can mean that employees' work is more

difficult and their quality of life is affected. Ultimately it can cause injuries to health.

When we use the word *"stress"* we usually mean negative stress.

Dr. Selye focused on the biological or physical effects of stress. Stress is currently said to be the feeling that a person experiences when the imposed demands on that person are greater than that person can handle or cope with. Also, the degree of stress experienced from stressors is determined by that particular person's perceptions, and past experiences, of various stressors.

Today, listening to and watching some of the news coverage about natural disasters, wars, etc., *can increase* our level of *stress* commensurate with our reaction to those events. And each day we may feel that the pressures of life—fears, frustrations within the family, interactions with neighbours, meeting deadlines, being on time for appointments, traffic snarls—all make our bodies feel as though they were facing threats—that is, the fight or flight response, the same reaction that our early ancestors experienced when facing physical danger.

The Stress Response

The *"stress response"* is our body's vital physical (body) or emotional (mind) *response* to fearful or exciting situations called stressors, which we encounter in daily living. This *"alarm system"* operates while the high-stress situation is being dealt with and subsequently subsides.

The stress response triggers the brain's hypothalamus, causing the nearby pituitary gland to release the hormone ACTH which prompts the adrenal glands atop the kidneys to secrete mainly adrenalin and cortisol hormones. The strength of the stress response is determined by the degree of excitement or fear that a person attaches to the stimulus (stressor). Secretion of stress hormones increases both oxygen in the blood and blood sugar. Result: more blood is sent to the muscles (increasing their strength and agility), the internal organs (thus reducing the risk of blood loss from superficial injuries), and the brain (resulting in a higher degree of awareness).

Acute Effects of Stress

The symptoms of Acute Stress include heartburn, headaches, profuse perspiration, insomnia, fatigue, and heart palpitations. Cortisol suppresses the immune system, thus putting a person at higher risk of infections. It reduces the rate of body repair and metabolism, and reduces the amount of nutrients available for the body. Adrenalin increases blood pressure and heart rate.

Chronic Effects of Stress

Chronic effects of stress include high blood pressure, stomach ulcers, weight gain, aching muscles, depression, insomnia, memory impairment, increased fear and anger, arthritis, osteoporosis, and cancer.

It may result in a higher percentage of stress-related illnesses, especially in genetically weak areas of the body. Recent studies indicate that some people who inherit a short stress-sensitive gene are more likely to become depressed than those who inherit the longer type of this gene.

Some Psychological Symptoms of Stress

- Anxiety
- Insomnia
- Fatigue
- Emotional numbness: no sadness, no pity (includes those people who have had very traumatic experiences, such as post-traumatic stress syndrome at any age).

Some Physical Symptoms of Stress

- Reduced immunity
- Increased aches and pains
- Increased perspiration
- Numbness in toes, fingers, and lips
- Anhedonia: the inability to feel joy or love
- Gastric and/or duodenal ulcers
- Chest pain, angina
- Higher blood pressure
- Thyroid problems
- Skin irritations such as athlete's foot, hives, acne, eczema, psoriasis
- Impotence

Major Factors Affecting Our Stress Response

- Employment/unemployment
- Emotional health
- Nutrition
- Use of illegal drugs/alcohol abuse
- The Relaxation Response

- After the mind realizes that our perceived danger, or threatening situation, is no longer present, our mind calms down, our body relaxes. Hormone levels, blood pressure, heart rate, and digestion all return to their previous normal levels.

- That is, our *"fight or flight response"* is followed by a *"relaxation response."*

Stress and Blood Pressure

Stan, the stress hormones cortisol, adrenaline, and ACTH, secreted during stress episodes, cause our blood vessels to contract and our heart to beat rapidly, resulting in temporarily increased blood pressure.

Apparently there is still no proof that stress alone, whether acute or chronic, causes long-term high blood pressure. However, stress-linked behaviours, such as overeating unhealthy foods, smoking, and drinking alcoholic beverages, may be contributing factors for long-term high blood pressure, heart attacks, and strokes.

Emotional conditions such as depression, anxiety, anger, and loneliness, alone, are not the direct cause of long-term high blood pressure.

However, the hormones produced during these emotional stress periods can lead to heart disease, because they damage arterial walls.

H. Lowering My Stress Level (part two)

The information below is taken from conversations with the above psychotherapist.

If I get worked up about things, in ordinary social contexts, it is not helpful! In most cases I need to tone down my fight or flight response by relaxation techniques or self-hypnosis. Unless, of course, I meet somebody who attacks me in a bar or on the street, then I must fight.

Under high threat, or fight or flight response, I automatically activate my pituitary gland at the base of the brain, and it secretes the adreno-cortico-tropic hormone (ACTH). My ACTH activates other glands to produce their specific hormones. The activated adrenal glands then secrete high levels of cortisol and adrenaline.

Therefore, toning down my fight or flight response is a good thing, because I don't need that surge of adrenaline and cortisol which moves me and motivates me, but too much increases my fear!

The other result of stress, other than fear, is anxiety! Anxiety also triggers the secretion of ACTH, and it activates the adrenal glands to secrete cortisol and adrenaline. A lot of cortisol was necessary in ancient man because it helped to heal wounds and reduce inflammation.

Now, I really have to "cool my jets", in other words, decrease my general fight or flight response and keep it limited over time, because long-term fear causes long-term elevated cortisol levels. This elevated cortisol level then kills off cells in my hippocampus, which is the part of my brain responsible for memory! This condition means that high levels of cortisol can cause my fear problem!

So I need to cool myself off with relaxation. No rushing is allowed.

I relax every chance I get; for example, while waiting in line at a bank. When walking, I walk in a way that the rhythm makes me relax. I can sit and think of nothing, which I seem to be able to do from time to time, automatically, which is actually okay for me.

It is true that, because of some of my childhood experiences, I have learned and can recall fearful memories. *Through hypnosis*, I am learning how to let go of all those negative memories; then I can go one step further, "*to let go*" of "*the letting go*" and I really "*let go*" when I "let go" of "*the letting go.*" Now I am letting my past hurtful experiences fall into "*a black hole*"!!!

It is now thought that the immune system is like a "*floating brain*," because the immune cells "*recognize*" old enemies they've seen before. The immune cells interact with the brain, because immune cells respond to serotonin and norepinephrine like the brain does.

Sometimes the immune system overreacts and causes the very problem it was trying to fix, in the sense that when it fights too hard, it causes collateral damage to whatever tissues it was fighting—for example, in the lungs, causing asthma!

Chronic high cortisol, on the other hand, can diminish the effectiveness of the immune system.

So, Stan, it is a delicate balance, the more at peace I am, the more likely my immune system is going to be neither overactive nor underactive. By being calm, I can avoid autoimmune diseases, like Crohn's disease, asthma, arthritis, etc. And chronic high levels of cortisol also increase cholesterol and body fat, which are risk factors for strokes and heart attacks.

Balance between all the hormones and neurotransmitters is the key. When they are all in a balanced state, that's when I feel the best. Meditation or self-hypnosis tend to shift everything into their balanced positions, and then everything works smoothly and wonderfully. That gives me a feeling of rejuvenation, loving peace, and joy that permeates my whole body, from the top of my head to the tips of my toes.

In this state of mind, I can rest so deeply, so completely, that when I awaken I feel totally refreshed, and that good feeling can linger through time and space. Even when I go to sleep, I feel at peace and I identify not necessarily with my thoughts and feelings, but simply with an awareness of peace deep within myself.

I have been uptight for years. This is usually increased by rushing to do too many things within a short period of time. Now I am slowly making successful attempts to diminish the frequency and amplitude of these hasty, agitated states. This attitude change takes time, but by achieving some degree of success now and then I have noticed somewhat less muscle tension in those moments when I am not a slave of the clock.

As I realize some success when the "*rushing urge arises,*" I feel that my "*no rush*" endeavour is beginning to succeed.

Rushing takes me away from the "*present.*" Therefore, I try not to cram in too many things at once when setting my goals for the day.

I have found that taking breaks is a wonderful way to avoid getting too rushed: e.g., tea break, coffee break, lunch break, a relaxing break, etc.

When I start to think that I have to increase the pace, I ask myself, "*Really, do I have to rush? Is it that important?*" If I am late for something, perhaps I can phone and say that I will be a little late.

Many people, like me, who rush, try to do too many things *at the same time.*

Focusing on doing one thing at a time is important, and I get satisfaction knowing that I get the job done.

I understand that rushing has a damaging effect on me because I lose my calmness, and my muscle tension increases. I know that I can live more peacefully instead of the hyper go, go, go, rushing attitude.

When I am after more productivity, I sometimes think of rushing to get more things done, but often I achieve more just by going at a normal pace. I think more clearly, my judgment is better, and I can laugh more.

Rushing takes me away from the present moment, and projects me into the future. I don't enjoy the *"rushing time,"* so I try to live in a non-rushing kind of way.

And at the end of the day, I achieve more than if I had been rushing all day. My mind likes to enjoy peace along the way; rushing steals the peace, and I want that peace. I can just refuse to rush and eventually it becomes a habit not to rush!

My anger is generally an attempt to control others to meet my needs. Fear lurks behind anger. Often my fear stems from a feeling of lack of control of myself or others.

I am now trying to accept my fear instead of fighting it. As I slowly learn to acknowledge my fear, I reduce my anxiety. I also find that I do not need anger to bring about change in a person or situation. Anger in such cases has only negative stress effects on my body. The harm done to myself by being angry is not easily reversible. By letting go, I actually gain control over myself.

I am becoming aware of potential anger and prepare for it. I now set realistic goals, and even small strides show that I am making progress.

I avoid saying *"should"* to people. It is self-destructive and is potentially harmful to relationships. When someone says *"You should ..."* to me, I feel that he or she *disapproves* of my statement, idea, or behaviour. The message from that person seems to be that only his or her opinion is *"The Absolute Truth"* or *"The Best Recommendation."*

Psychotherapist:

Normally when the stress situation has ended, the steroid levels go down and the immune system returns to normal, so they have a kind of reciprocal relationship. In other words, the steroids inhibit the immune system which is a good thing if you have, say, asthma, or multiple sclerosis, or rheumatoid arthritis. You can use steroids externally to decrease the activity of the immune system when it gets overzealous. When the immune system is weak, you can reduce the stress which then decreases steroids. The steroids allow the immune system to revive its strength. So you can see how the systems are all tied up, one with the other.

Apparently there are *"feedback mechanisms"* between the autonomic nervous system and the central nervous system, in the sense if you have anxious thoughts they turn up the adrenalin which comes from the adrenal cortex and then gets your body ready for the *"fight or flight"* response, which is very important when you are in an *"urgent"* situation. It is a wonderful thing to then have extra energy, and the adrenalin diverts the blood supply to the muscles so that you can take *"fight or flight"* action.

And, of course, a lot of these connections between systems have grown over many years of evolution, so even imaginary fear can result in activation of the immune system. And so when you get rid of the imaginary fear, you realize that it is only imaginary. The minute that imaginary thought is realized, and influences your hypothalamus and all the hormones from the pituitary, all the hormones from the target organs, including the thyroid and the adrenal glands, resume normal functioning.

Also, emotions are run by neuropeptides, which can influence the endocrine system, which can also influence the autonomic nervous system. So now you begin to see the systems are all "*talking*" to one another.

When you are relaxed, it is easier to imagine a huge picture of a boardroom and four members of the various systems all talking to one another and agreeing on either revving up the immune system, revving it down, revving up the fight or flight response or revving it down, and deciding that chronic stress is not a good thing. And deciding when you come to see the psychotherapist that expectancy, positive expectancy, can even improve the perception of feeling, neurotransmitters of various systems in your brain change, especially the dopamine which seems to run the expectancy part of things.

So there you have the neurotransmitter dopamine, affecting the nervous system. Feeling good changes the perception of pain in your feet. And probably expectancy decreases the steroids and therefore your blood pressure, which is part of the autonomic nervous system. And so, if you can, imagine, Bud, a boardroom, where the directors (systems) are all talking and agreeing on various principles of doing the fight or flight response if necessary, but not on a chronic basis. In other words, between urgent problems, and the ability to relax is very wonderful. It tones down everything, so that you have a normal cortisol level for example, and your immune system functions very well, thank you very much. And you have a normal thyroid flow, which allows your heart to beat regularly, but not fast. And round and round you go, for all the systems that we know.

But think of a boardroom, Bud, where there are various discussions going on, how to handle different situations, like how to handle foot pain, is to have positive expectancy for one thing, and another thing is to know to be absorbed in various things, like reading or writing. Being creative like you are doing with your project, being absorbed in it, you forget about your body for a while, let it heal. We know now that things can heal when we didn't think they could heal—the brain can heal through neurogenesis, the heart can heal through proper diet, better than we ever thought.

It is better to relax and not push too hard. There is much more information about being gentle and soothing with yourself. Of course, our famous saying is that *"There is no need to rush."* Now just be effortless, smooth, and flowing, and all your systems will work their best, and that means that the people in boardroom are all getting along famously!

Stan, aside from the above gem-quality information, this psychotherapist recommended this for reducing stress on a daily basis:

- Inhale & exhale deeply at the belt level, ten times three times per day.

- Write down three positive experiences or benefits that you are happy to have.

Some Examples of the Systems and How They Interact

During the reproductive years, people seek mates. The hormones of the endocrine system influence the central nervous system. During the sexual act, erection and ejaculation of the penis are operated by the autonomic nervous system.

When students write exams their stress level increases. Stress of the central nervous system influences the endocrine system by increasing cortisol production which decreases the immune system function, resulting in viral infections or colds.

The four systems—autonomic nervous system, central nervous system, endocrine system, and immune system—overlap. The best way to understand it is as four overlapping circles. For example, if you see a bear on the trail, you get a sympathetic response of fight or flight, and your endocrine system secretes adrenalin and raises the cortisol level so the main part of the sympathetic nervous system diverts the blood flow to the muscles, and for the moment takes blood away from the visceral organs and the cortisone increases, which is an anti-inflammatory response.

So, if you are injured in some way, the cortisone would calm down the injury so that you could continue your fight or flight response. So there you see the nervous system interacting with the endocrine system, and, if you step back, you'll see the central nervous system and then the autonomic nervous system interacting with the endocrine system with a cortisol increase.

The immune system starts to kick into gear because it realizes that there is some threat to the integrity of the body. It increases the potential for the immune system response, so, having seen the bear, it starts responses in all your systems, including, of course, the genes, and turns them on and off. That is, certain genes that make the proteins to supply the endocrine system with neurotransmitters.

H. Retraining My Brain

The information below is taken from conversations with the psychotherapist.

Stan, now that you've read about and are aware of my experiences of shame, fears, and a few betrayals, I think you'll agree that my brain requires "retraining."

As a newborn, I was physically complete. At this stage of life, my brain was on standby, waiting for new experiences.

As a very young child, the quality of the nurturing experiences I had affected my thinking processes. It is said that the brains of children who are deprived of a stimulating environment do not develop to their full potential.

For example, when children are repeatedly abused or traumatized, their fears become somewhat fixed. Traumatized children, like me, continue to exhibit fear, even in the absence of the frightening experiences. Generally, such children develop high levels of stress hormones.

I wonder if my upbringing had some bearing on my periods of sadness and despair to the point of being disruptive to my social functioning, and regular activities of daily living. Or is it a combination of the above, plus my genetic makeup? It really doesn't matter. What is important is that I continue, in regular small steps, to overcome my shame, fears, and anxiety.

My Action Plan

- My learned fears are stored in, and are triggered by, the amygdala and anxieties by the striaterminalis, both working automatically in my brain. To diminish these fears, and anxieties, I am taking small, but repeated specific actions.

- Examples: Some people take part in public speaking to overcome their fear of public speaking. Actors practise acting to overcome their stage fright. Both activities overcome fear with active repetition.

- Research has shown that we can have only one thought at a time, although at times that one thought can be interfered with by obsessive thoughts. However, when I focus on the most important task first, with blinders on, I can lose myself in the task until completion.

- By doing tasks in order of their priority, I can make them appear less overwhelming. By taking appropriate breaks, I can help to ease my mind and work more efficiently.

- Positive reinforcement: When small goals are accomplished, or even exceeded, I feel a little happier, because success triggers the dopamine reward system. Small successes make it more likely that I will succeed again—and in more difficult tasks!

- As we learn information, neural circuits grow new brain connections. As I use my spare time to keep learning, I cause neurons to grow. This phenomenon is called neurogenesis, the formation of new brain cells.

- Taking bigger risks: The brain wants to play it safe and survive. It's my amygdala that stores my fearful emotions and keeps me from doing things in which I might fail. Also, the amygdala, when stimulated, not only triggers fear, it can also trigger neural circuits that create anger and feelings of revenge. I can boost my self-confidence by taking appropriate risks.

- Our primitive social dominance system creates a "necessary" desire for status. Once needed for survival, this "necessary" status desire can lead to hate, discrimination, exclusion, and even war. Our best bet is to join groups of people who are compassionate, friendly, and sympathetic towards all people.

- Our brain's amygdala wants to react instantly, automatically, to trigger anger and revenge. It's good to be assertive but not aggressive.

Stan, I now go into a hypnotic trance, listening to the psychotherapist talk about the brain's frontal lobes + the amygdala interactions:

Psychotherapist:

The brain's frontal lobes, particularly the left frontal lobe, have to do with the taming of the amygdala; its fear and anger responses in particular.

Bud, you can build up the connections from the left frontal lobe to the amygdala like saying to yourself, *"That's my overreaction to that particular problem. I don't have to catastrophize, there's no need to fear."*

In a kind of way, the frontal lobe says to the amygdala, *"Don't worry, baby, I'll look after you, I know when to handle things. I have faith that somehow, some way, I'll handle whatever comes my way."*

The amygdala says, *"Okay then, I'll relax, but mind you, you know that I'll keep on watching."*

The frontal lobe says back, *"Well, yes, you can keep watching and I need you."*

It's very important to keep that balance of fear and rage, so that neither needlessly slides into extreme fear or extreme anger.

An example of this idea of the frontal lobe taming the amygdala, with regard to, for example, depression or hate, is the frontal lobes of Buddhists monks. They become quite developed because they meditate on compassion, and loving kindness. They don't even kill an insect. They are compassionate to all people. Every sentient (able to sense or feel) being, which includes insects, animals, and of course humans, they cultivate that, and they include compassion towards themselves as well. They also meditate on loving kindness, you know, the random acts of kindness, kind of thing.

The Dalai Lama talks extensively about how if you have a mindset of compassion and loving kindness, and you cultivate that mindset in meditation, over and over and over, then when you are faced with events in the world that could incite anger, hatred, or even violence, you meet them with compassion and loving kindness, because that's the way you've programmed your brain, by training it.

Think of all the ways that you can be compassionate, and all the ways you have been compassionate. Just the little things you do, saying "*hello*" to somebody, and grasping his or her hand, and as you recognize and appreciate each other, in the present moment, as kind human beings. You have a moment of acknowledgement, which is an act of kindness, loving kindness.

You can be compassionate when you help friends who are sick, or struggling. You can be compassionate when you talk to somebody who is distressed.

You can be compassionate to yourself, when you become a really, really, solid good friend to yourself, self-soothing. It allows you to become compassionate, and loving toward other people. That kind of training changes your brain! You'll notice it because you'll react to the same old event in a different way. You'll know you've re-patterned the synapses between your amygdala and your frontal lobes and vice versa.

One of the ways that I train myself is by visualizing myself being compassionate to myself, and to other people, seeing it, feeling it, deep in my bones. Sometimes, I just feel more loving towards the world, and people pick up on it. It takes time, years of practice.

I can have "*aha moments*" when I realize that one aspect of my personality is talking to the other aspect of my personality. Sometimes metaphors are a wonderful way to build up the connections.

An example I, Bud, am sitting on a park bench, and I am at my current age. I see this young chap walking towards me. I seem to know who he is, and I find out that is the Young Me! The Young Me who is lonely and scared, and perhaps tired and depressed, having been verbally abused by six family members whom I have forgiven. I get close to that Young Me, and that Older Me gives him a big hug. I say to him, *"I'll look after you, kid."* That just warms my heart and warms the Young Me's heart and sets up whole different patterns. I can, being in the "æ" alter the past in significant ways, because I am different now. I can rewrite my attitude towards the past, and make it sit in a different way!

I can do this most efficiently by taking the time to r-e-l-a-x, and I drift into a very, very peaceful state. And–the–deeper–I–go–the–more–comfortable–I–can–be–the–more–comfortable–I–am–the–deeper–I–can–go–every muscle–every–nerve– r-e-l-a-x-e-d …

I take my time. I don't need to rush! I just enjoy how time s-l-o-w-s down.

When I rush, I start the stress response, and the pituitary-hypothalamic-adrenal axis gets lit up with high cortisol levels, which aggravates all kinds of things.

So I want to r-e-l-a-x, and live life *"hypnotically."* And every time I feel stressed, I take a moment to drift into a wonderful, restful trance. Relaxing works and it is all up to me, and it belongs to me.

Chapter 14 – Forgiving

The information below is taken from conversations with a psychotherapist.

A famous act of forgiveness occurred when Pope John Paul II went to the prison where his would-be assassin was being held. The Pope said to this man, *"I forgive you."*

Stan, you and I, and perhaps everyone else in the world, have been hurt by the words or actions of other people at some stage. These emotional wounds leave us with lasting feelings of resentment, anger, and even thoughts of harmful revenge.

Psychotherapist:

If we dwell on these emotional wounds of the past, though, we are the ones who continue to suffer, and often in silence.

Healing these emotional wounds can be achieved, in time, by adopting or developing a *"forgiving attitude"*. When we embrace forgiveness we experience greater emotional well-being and we can gradually diminish our resentful, unforgiving attitude.

Forgiving is a decision taken by people to release themselves from the thoughts and feelings that tie them to the offences perpetrated against them. Forgiveness can reduce the strength of the emotional feelings that result from these offences, so that living a happier life in the *"precious present"* is possible.

Practising forgiveness can lead to a greater understanding of the perpetrator, and perhaps help the victim develop some compassion or empathy for the person who was their tormentor.

Acts of torment can remain with a person for life, but forgiveness can diminish their impact. A person who is the victim can forgive the perpetrator without forgiving the hurtful act.

Stan, in order for me to diminish the suffering I endured because of past conditioned responses to shame, fear, broken promises, and other sources of unhappiness, I must reduce, and perhaps eliminate, my current feelings of resentment.

- The only way for me to decrease my resentments is for me to forgive each person for the pain and anxiety that he or she has caused me, in both the recent and the distant past.

- I must repeat the forgiveness process over and over, until nothing is left of my feelings of resentment, which hinder my potential abilities.

- I have been wasting energy by thinking about these hurts of the recent and distant past. This psychological pain cannot be solved with repeated thoughts about them, and I need to harvest the energy I have been wasting. This recovered energy is slowly becoming available for me to use as I follow through on my new constructive changes!!!

Some action steps for acquiring forgiveness:

- I imagine a certain person while I sit in a comfortable chair, and pay attention to my breathing.

- Then I visualize that person, further and further away from me, placing that person at a less threatening distance.

- As I feel more relaxed, I address the person by name and talk to them in a normal tone of voice. I can focus my attention in the *"present moment"* without wandering off into past memories.

- As I call out to the person by name, I begin to reduce my resentments, anger, and frustrations, all of which I have kept bottled up in the past.

- By so doing, I begin to release those negative energies and thoughts about that person, without hurting that person.

- I let myself feel the experience of accusing that person in the "*present*," and when I feel that, I do not continue.

- I break off the fantasy conversation, perhaps until later or until the following day. This step puts me in touch with my resentment, as I explain to that person exactly how I feel!!!

- Now I provide the opportunity for the imagined person to reply to what I have said. My attention and energy are directed into listening to what is being said to me!!!

- I become engaged in this back-and-forth conversation until there are no words left unsaid between us.

- This fantasy dialogue demands a great deal of my energy, because I am still learning how to listen to a person whom I resent.

- When I find it too difficult to imagine how the other person replies, I discontinue the acting and try again when I feel calmer.

- When I am able to engage that person again in this "*fantasy dialogue*," I try to keep it going back and forth until I feel that it is finished. As mentioned before, this technique demands a great deal of energy, because I am de-conditioning myself from past resentments. Therefore, when I feel exhausted, or when the dialogue lapses into silence, I stop.

What are the benefits of forgiving?

- The act of forgiveness is an expression of growth in the human personality. I find that it allows me to understand and acknowledge that many persons in my life have also been affected, in unfortunate ways, by their past conditioning. But despite their learned negative behaviour, they are doing the best they can.

- In the act of forgiving another person for their "*misdeeds*" and that person's real or imagined limitations, I come to understand the meaning of compassion. I am beginning to understand that each one of us has karma (karma is an action seen as bringing upon oneself inevitable results, good or bad, either in this life or in reincarnation, if this is your belief).

- I, like most of us, am imperfect, incomplete, and that is perhaps why we humans have a need for each other. To get in touch with that realization, I need to invest a great amount of creative energy. This step can also demand "*role playing*" on my part. This is where I try on new behaviours for size, and learn how forgiveness actually works. Unfortunately, my efforts to de-condition my resentments can flounder, and my energies can begin to wane.

- I will not grow and change just by thinking about change. And I cannot learn how to forgive just by thinking about it. I can learn what forgiveness is only through the act of forgiving!!! The closer I get to being capable of saying, "*I forgive you*"—in fantasy or in person—the more likely I am to become a forgiving person in "*the present moment.*"

My psychotherapist addressed the issue of forgiveness by using hypnosis on me. As I went into a hypnotic trance, he responded to pertinent points from my past.

Example: In order to keep me in line, my mother would often threaten to call "*Mr. Skinner*" over to "*skin me alive*" if I misbehaved. Perhaps this concept of instilling fear into children to encourage better behaviour was learned by my mother from her parents.

Psychotherapist:

Let's start with your mom who told you at times that Mr. Skinner would come and *"skin you alive"* if you misbehaved. You know when we talked about that, in the sense that parents, especially young parents like your mom, weren't taught much and they used fear to control their kids. It certainly worked in the sense that the metaphor of Mr. Skinner and being *"skinned alive"* were taken very literally by little children. Kids are very literal, and they think in terms of really being *"skinned!"*

So you have to think about your mother's limitations in raising children, and say to yourself, *"Well she didn't understand that fear is not a good motivator, and she probably didn't understand how literally kids think."*

And so her lack of understanding, you know, ended up causing you fear. But to let go of that fear, finally, is to forgive her. You must understand that she was uninformed of better ways for training her children.

Example: Often, while I sat in my highchair with my parents seated at the kitchen table across from me, they would have heated arguments. My father had once been a corporal—during peacetime—in the Austrian army, and his loud commanding voice frightened me. After each argument was over, my father would leave in anger, slamming the back door behind him!

Psychotherapist:

The next point is that your father would use a loud commanding voice. Again, you know, it's the same old thing of a loud voice causing fear in the kid, and slamming the door is a power move, a move out of anger. It's a move on the part of your dad to gain control rather than talking to you. You know, human to human, he just wanted to get a response through fear.

Example: When sent to the corner store on my tricycle, I had to pass Petri's fenced-in vicious dog. I can still visualize the dog's thick saliva, stretching between its teeth as it snarled and barked, and that memory is now entrenched indelibly in my brain's amygdala. Somehow the dog managed to bite two people, and when the police were alerted, they shot the dog while it was still in the yard (they took no chances in capturing the dangerous dog for execution elsewhere).

Psychotherapist:

I can remember being scared by a dog just as you were. In fact, the dog did bite me. It was actually put down eventually, but I used to gird my loins going past the house where the dog would sit on the porch and growl. He would show his teeth at me. The damn thing finally did take a chunk out of me. But that dog actually, in the sense that it had some kind of a feeling, that if anyone came near the property, he was protecting the property, and it got out of hand. Fortunately, they found out that it did not have distemper, which is a good thing for me to find out. I guess you have to forgive the dog, and the people who owned the dog, and finally, let go of that fear.

Example: Being the only one in our family of seven who could not read, I felt very inadequate and ashamed. Not knowing any better, I sat for hours on end in front of the bookcase, trying to read both English and Cyrillic script. Eventually, I asked my mother to teach me how to read. She replied, "*You will have to wait until you go to school.*" Therefore, I continued attempting to teach myself to read. I believe that my failure at this led to initiating my depression.

Psychotherapist:

It's too bad that your mom didn't help you to read. She could have nurtured you in a more meaningful way, and helped you translate those "*squiggly lines.*" Again, you have to forgive your mother for not having known better methods for raising children.

Example: Prior to attending school and for almost 15 years thereafter, my mother and older sister Tory teased me because one of my playmates was a girl! In my later years, even though I desired female companionship, I resisted because of the thought of a family member, or even a family friend, learning of such a relationship. This early negative, emotional sadistic teasing later led me to develop a drastic plan: If I ever made a woman pregnant, I would immediately change my name and move to a different location. Now, I realize—too late—that procreation is a normal issue between consenting partners.

Psychotherapist:

Then your mom and your older sister Tory teased you because one of your playmates was a girl!

What is teasing? Teasing often has a *"barb"* in it or a *"hook,"* and again it's sort of a power move on the part of the teasers to feel better than ... You know, if the object of the teasing is embarrassed and hurt, they feel more powerful. But then you can be more powerful in the end ... by forgiving your mother and Tory for their silly moves that they made when you were young.

Through the years, hopefully, especially now that you can forgive your mother and Tory, you may be more and more comfortable talking to women of all shapes and sizes, personalities. In fact, in group situations, you are often quite conversant with other ladies in a group, as I recall.

The teasing about making a woman pregnant, and changing your name, and moving to a different location: Teasing, I've read about, is a form of, just like you say, sadism. Again, it's how the teaser gets to feel better. And it is an insecurity operation in the sense that they (the teasers) need to stand on other people's shoulders to feel better. So understanding that in a deep sense and understanding that we are all insecure, you begin to forgive the teaser. And actually feel sorry for them, in a way that they have to resort to that method to gain any sense of self-esteem.

Example: Soon after my 16th birthday, I obtained a summer job at the CNR Stores Department, unloading lumber from boxcars. In view of my turning over my endorsed cheques to my parents, I asked my mother if I could be compensated with a pair of skis for the upcoming winter season. Her answer was a definite yes!!! I told my friends that this winter I would finally be able to join them for skiing at the large CNR snow-covered coal piles. Winter arrived, and I asked my mother for the promised skis. Now, the answer was no!!! My sister Vera, four years my senior, was standing next to our mother. She added, "*You are too skinny to ski anyway*". Mother and daughter turned to face each other, each smirking, as I watched in deep disappointment and shame.

Psychotherapist:

Then the broken promise about the skis that your mother promised and what did her promise mean? It didn't mean that she was going to fulfill it, and then to top it all off, probably she felt guilty about not fulfilling it.

So again, Vera using an insult, sarcasm, and teasing put you in a shamed position. It's a cheap way to find a sense of worth, so forgive her and move on.

Example: My two brothers, Joe and Ted, bestowed upon me two pet names by which they addressed me: either "*Booby*" or "*Asshole*." Their closest friends also addressed me as "*Boob*" or "*Booby*," and "*Asshole*."

Psychotherapist:

Then Booby and Asshole, you know, are names which like "*sticks and stones can break my bones but names will never hurt me*." That is what you have to remember, Bud. We used to say that as kids, because lots of times we'd be teased by other kids or "*bullied*," and you'd yell that back to them. So in your mind you can yell that back, and then when you do, you can let it go. Because really to treat yourself well, your psychotherapist is saying let it go, Bud, and then you can even let go of that letting go! And let it sink into oblivion!!!

Example: Without my asking for it, my two brothers put forth this fantastic offer! I was told to quit my plywood mill job, make a small investment, renovate interiors of several West End houses, and receive one third of the profits!!! Ted added, *"You will then have enough money to go back to university and even buy a car!"* One house, at 1648 Davie Street (the current location of London Drugs), was in my name only. Eventually, my promised one-third profit share dropped dramatically to one used colour TV, which I declined (see R86, in Remembering). A mutual friend, Adam, once asked me, *"Why do your brothers talk about you that way?"* Without asking Adam what my brothers said about me, I replied, "I don't know." Adam replied emphatically, *"They want to suppress you, put you down!!!"*

Psychotherapist:

When your brothers cheated you on the profits, they were taking advantage of your naivety. If there is a heaven, I am sure that they will pay their dues. There again, putting you down to put themselves up—what a dishonourable way to gain a sense of worth.

Example: My brother Ted and his wife purchased a house in White Rock. Soon after during a telephone conversation, and in full knowledge that my wife and I were renting a one-bedroom apartment in the West End of Vancouver, Ted announced, *"You really have only one room there, and the only place you can read is in the can."*

Psychotherapist:

Then your brother made fun of your one-bedroom apartment. But you know, at the end of the day, Bud, it's not material goods it is your inner soul that matters. You can take comfort that you've been a good soul through your life, and you haven't lashed back, and you can let it go—forgive! Maybe you don't want to forget, but you can forgive!

But you want to remember, of course, the lesson that when someone anytime does anything along those lines, you just stand up and say, *"F**K YOU!"* How's that?

Example: On occasion, in company, when a person paid me a compliment, one of my brothers would reply, "*He's not so smart.*"

Psychotherapist:

Your brothers would say, "*He's not so smart,*" and they did say it in company, which is a cheap shot!!!

Example: Miss McKeller, my grade 3 teacher, was kind to me. She allowed me to assist students who needed help with arithmetic and problem solving. Perhaps Miss McKeller's benevolent nature induced in me a less fearful, calmer frame of mind, because my report would sometimes rate three, out of a class of thirty students.

Psychotherapist:

Thank God for people like Miss McKeller, your third grade teacher, who asked you to help other kids and made you less fearful. Now you were number three, what an honour!

Example: A dance instructor once said to me, "*Someone must have been very mean to you.*" I was stunned at this comment. I repeated the dance instructor's words to a psychotherapist, who replied, "*Yes, they can tell!*"

Psychotherapist:

The dance instructor, you know, probably picked up on your non-verbal reticence. You know, people who have been "*put down*" do have less freedom about their bodies.

Now you can enjoy j-u-s-t f-e-e-l-i-n-g f-r-e-e.

Example: Having been raised in a verbally abusive family, I am not surprised that I learned or copied sadistic behaviour (see R62 in Remembering).

Stan, the following analogy may be overly simplistic, but it will illustrate my point. Many people claim that "seeing is believing." Approximately 10% of an iceberg floating in water is what we actually see, and this can be equated to what we apparently see in a person's behaviour. The unseen 90% of an iceberg can be equated to the unseen, or learned, experiences which cause a person's 90% "seen" behaviour.

So, Stan, this analogy may help many people to be aware of the important impact of the formative years, or "unseen" learned experiences, on the development of human behaviour.

Psychotherapist:

You can't choose the family that you were raised in, but you can transcend their belief systems and believe in treating people respectfully and honouring people. In your transcendence, transcend any patterns created by the earlier years.

But forgiveness, Bud, is a combination of understanding other people's ignorance and developing a thicker skin and being tougher.

One of the toughest things for anyone to do is to let go of the hurt and pain, to move on and forgive. In a sense, you understand that most of the negativity coming from other people is out of their low self-esteem, and their fear!!! They want to be better ... it makes them less fearful of life and so forth. So they are acting out of weakness, rather than strength. In your life, Bud, I'm sure you met people who were strong and they didn't have to tease, they didn't have to belittle, they didn't have to "*dis (discount) people,*" as kids say now. They respect you and you respect them.

Even in the Lord's prayer, "*We forgive those who trespass against us.*" That is how important forgiveness is as part of the Lord's Prayer. Possibly this part of the Lord's Prayer refers to the fact that we probably hurt others and do not know it.

So you are asking for forgiveness for yourself, too, which helps you forgive others.

Forgiveness is like a cleansing feeling, like having a shower, like taking next steps. It is like being able to feel free, it's like weights falling off your shoulders, it's a lightness based on a deep understanding of human nature. So just bask in the comfort zone, Bud, where you just "*Forgive those who trespass against you*"—really relaxed, so relaxed, more than you've been f-o-r a l-o-n-g, l-o-n-g, t-i-m-e. In that r-e-l-a-x-e-d state it is easier to forgive, as you can imagine yourself as a person who is a forgiving person who can move on, let go of past hurts, free yourself of the burden. As you do so, your inner part of yourself feels stronger, and you can go as d-e-e-p-l-y as you need to go, find that comfort d-e-e-p within you.

Chapter 15 – Defining Mental Illness and History of Depression

Defining Mental Illness is taken as noted. History of Depression from conversations with a psychotherapist.

Since ancient times, some people have suffered from symptoms of depressive illness.

Around 2000 b.c., physicians in Rome and in Greek cities prescribed rest for depressed patients. They also found that waters in the spas of northern Italy helped to calm these disturbed people. Much later, these waters were found to contain dissolved lithium salt compounds. Lithium carbonate is a drug now used orally to prevent or treat schizophrenia and similar psychiatric disorders.

About 1,600 years ago, the Greco-Roman treatments for these unfortunate depressed people became less humane. It was thought that the devil had control of their minds, and some were chained, bled, given potions, or killed. Fortunately, physicians in the Islamic countries continued the older, more humane *"conventional treatments"* of rest and bathing.

After the 1700s, the more humane original treatments for mental disorders were re-established—for example, bed rest and isolation from the public—which helped to calm patients.

In the early 1900s, Dr. Sigmund Freud, and others, developed the psychoanalytic technique. This concept was founded on the belief that depressive illnesses were initiated by early childhood traumas that had not been adequately resolved—hence a couch for patient relaxation, and talk therapy between patient and psychoanalyst to explore traumas of the patient's past.

Up until about the 1950s, patients were usually placed in institutions. Barbiturates, bromides, narcotics, and sedation drugs were the conventional medications. Along with these medications, warm baths, shock therapies using either drugs or electric shock, and prefrontal lobotomies were performed.

With the development of antipsychotic and antidepressant drugs, less intense electroconvulsive therapy was used. The mentally ill were no longer institutionalized. Psychiatrists, psychologists, and other mental health providers became community based, which has helped to eliminate the stigma of mental illness.

Mental illness is found in people from all levels of society. The following is a short list who some claim, have suffered from a mental illness:

- Abraham Lincoln (16th U.S. President)
- Adolph Hitler (German dictator)
- Ernest Hemingway (U.S. novelist, short-story writer, & journalist)
- Eugene O'Neill (U.S. playwright)
- Isaac Newton (English scientist, mathematician, & physicist)
- John Keats (English poet)

- Joseph Stalin (Russian dictator)
- Leo Tolstoy (Russian author)
- Ludwig Beethoven (composer)
- Michelangelo (Italian artist)
- Napoleon Bonaparte (French dictator)
- Vincent Van Gogh (artist)
- Virginia Woolf English novelist, essayist, & critic)
- Winston Churchill (British prime minister)

Depression

From time to time, everyone experiences the pain of unhappiness because of what we perceive as setbacks or losses. And these unhappy feelings are usually appropriate. However, when a low mood persists on a daily basis for two weeks, this may indicate that the person is in a state of depression.

Symptoms of depression:

- A depressed or irritable mood on most days.
- Reduced pleasure or interest in most daily activities.
- Significant decrease or increase in appetite with subsequent weight loss or weight gain.
- Insomnia or excessive sleepiness.
- Agitated feelings or retardation with a sense of being slowed down.
- Feelings of worthlessness or inappropriate guilt most of the time.
- Fatigue, with daily low level of energy.
- Reduced ability to concentrate or make decisions most of the time.

- Repeated thoughts of death or suicide.
- Avoiding other people
- Lowered sex drive
- Deep feelings of sadness or grief

Causes of Depression

The exact causes of depressive illnesses are still not known, although it is known to be due to interactions between psychological and neurological components, and can run in families. Studies show biological changes in the brains of people with clinical depression, especially in neurotransmitters which are involved in transmitting signals between brain cells and neurons. The main neurotransmitters are serotonin, dopamine, and noradrenalin. They regulate emotion and mood, plus hormonal disturbances in the function of sleep. Another concept is that depression may be caused by an array of genes rather than one gene.

Psychological factors such as stressful lifestyle, social isolation, early childhood traumas, job or financial loss, and retirement can also trigger depression.

Some authorities on depression claim it is caused by endogenous (*endo* = within + genesis = origin) or internal causes. An opposite school of thought claims that depression originates because of ectogenous (*ecto* = external + genesis = origin), or external causes.

Complexity of Depression

Depression is categorized into several major types, and each major type has its own sub-groups:

- *Bipolar* disorder generally describes people whose moods range from a clinical depression state to a highly elevated mood state—that is, a mixture of a depressed state of mind, and alternately, an elevated state of mind. Each depressive mood state and each elevated mood state vary widely in their intensity and duration. The person's bipolar mood swings are called "*cycling.*"

- The bipolar spectrum is the range of depressive diseases ranging from bipolar disorder to clinical (or unipolar, or major depression) depression. The depression referred to here is not the everyday feeling of being somewhat "*down*" or "*depressed.*"

- *Unipolar* affective disorder/major depressive disorder/clinical depression is the repeated experiences of depression alone, without the occurrence of elevated (mania) episodes. It is a state of sadness that is severe enough to disrupt the person's social functioning and daily living activities.

- Clinical depression may occur as a single episode, or recurrent episodes throughout a person's lifetime. It is said to be the leading cause of disability throughout the world. According to the World Health Organization, clinical depression is expected to become the second leading cause of disability worldwide, after heart disease, by the year 2020.

- *Dysthymia* is a depressive mood disorder where the person does not experience full enjoyment or pleasure in life. It continues for about two years and may or may not prevent a person from functioning well in daily activities. Dysthymia sufferers have fairly mild daily symptoms. However, over their lifetime, dysthymics experience high suicide rates, work problems, and social isolation. Typically, dysthymia lasts longer than an episode of clinical (or major) depression. Dysthymics have:

- o low energy levels or fatigue
- o sleep disturbances (either increased or decreased sleeping)
- o low self-esteem
- o a feeling of hopelessness
- o problems making decisions

- *Dysphoria* is the opposite of euphoria. Dysphorics feel mental discomfort, restlessness, sadness, and depression. Some are gender dysphorics, not satisfied with their sex or gender. People with bipolar disorder often suffer from "*dysphoria highs*" when they are feeling "*up*."

- *Postpartum depression*, also known as postnatal depression (post = after + natal = birth), is a form of clinical depression that can affect women after the birth of a child. However, men can suffer from similar, albeit less severe, emotions after the birth of a child. It can be easy to confuse postpartum depression with the normal overwhelming hormonal and physical effects of childbirth which are known to trigger emotional symptoms. Most postpartum women have a mild, fleeting, lowered mood, which lasts from hours to several days, such as headache, crying, irritability, sleeplessness, and impaired concentration—this is not postpartum depression. True postpartum depression usually occurs shortly after the birth of the child, and the degree of depression can range from very mild depression to severe psychotic depression. Postpartum depression symptoms are present for approximately one month and, like clinical depression, require professional treatment.

Defining Mental Illness

We can all be *"sad"* or *"blue"* at times in our lives. We have all seen movies about a madman and his crime spree, with the underlying cause of mental illness. We sometimes even make jokes about people being crazy or nuts, even though we know that we shouldn't. We have all had some exposure to mental illness, but do we really understand it or know what it is? Many of our preconceptions are incorrect. A mental illness can be defined as a health condition that changes a person's thinking, feelings, or behavior (or all three) and that causes the person distress and difficulty in functioning.

As with many diseases, mental illness is severe in some cases and mild in others. Individuals who have a mental illness don't necessarily look like they are sick, especially if their illness is mild. Other individuals may show more explicit symptoms such as confusion, agitation, or withdrawal.

In fact, the surgeon general reports that mental illnesses are so common that few U.S. families are untouched by them.

Excerpts Taken From: National Institutes of Health (US); Biological Sciences Curriculum Study. NIH Curriculum Supplement Series [Internet]. National Institutes of Health (US); 2007

Mental illness or mental disorders include:

- Anxiety disorders, including panic disorder, obsessive-compulsive disorder, post-traumatic stress disorder and phobias
- Bipolar disorder
- Depression

- Mood disorders
- Psychotic disorders, including schizophrenia
- There are many causes of mental disorders:
    - Your genes and family history may play a role
    - Your life experiences, such as stress or history of abuse, may also matter.
    - Biological factors can also be part of the cause. A traumatic brain injury can lead to a mental disorder.
    - A mother's exposure to viruses or toxic chemicals while pregnant may play a part.
    - Other factors may increase your risk, such as use of illegal drugs or having a serious medical condition like cancer.
    - Medications and counseling can help many mental disorders.

From: http://www.nlm.nih.gov/medlineplus/mentaldisorders.html

You can listen for free, to an internationally known depression expert Dr. Michael Yapko, at www.youtube. Dr. Yapko's books are sold on www.amazon.com.

One psychotherapist told me that he met Dr. Michael Yapko, a California based psychologist and world renowned depression expert.

Yapko is the author of 13 books on hypnosis and treating depression. His books have been translated in nine languages. He was also chosen to write the section on "Treating Depression" "Clinical Depression" and "Brief

Therapy" for the Encyclopedia Britannica Medical and Health Annals."

Taken from: Wikipedia the free encyclopedia

Chapter 16 - The Power of Positive Thought in Combating Depression

The information below is taken from conversations with a psychotherapist.

If you think positively you can start the C-fos gene (induced growth factor or vascular endothelial growth factor D) going, and researchers can measure it. That has an influence in terms of, for example, blood flow to the frontal lobes of the brain.

- In depression, the blood flow to the frontal lobes of the brain is diminished. With psychotherapy, after a number of weeks the blood flow improves in the frontal lobes! (You can see this in a *PET scan.)

- Don't fall into the trap of thinking in terms of catastrophes that you cannot control. For example, I'm hoping that the weather will be nice tomorrow but I'm not going to get too obsessed about it because I can't control the weather—who can? It's like a serenity prayer. You don't worry about things that are out of your control, you control things that you can control. Those kinds of thoughts can actually change blood flow, but how does the blood flow in the frontal lobes change?

- Well, the genes' on-off switches work in such a way that they produce proteins that affect the metabolism of cells or neurons. So every change in the body is somehow monitored by the genes. Researchers once thought that genes just sat there and did their job by determining hair colour, eye colour, etc. Wrong!!! They are dynamic, vigorously active! Genes are constantly changing! And genes will change in reaction to hormones that change, for example, if you have a lot of stress and you produce a lot of cortisol [internal secretion from the adrenal glands which is a stress response], and if you have more than enough cortisol, it will destroy the cells in the hippocampus, so your memory is impaired if you have enough stress. Phew!

- If you de-stress yourself, practise relaxation and so forth, your level of cortisol goes down, which improves the cells in your hippocampus, which also improves your immune system, because cortisol also suppresses your immune system. And it is all done through your genes!

- Our genes are dynamic, so our thinking patterns can have an influence on our genes! Now that's hopeful, because we can, to some extent, control our thinking patterns.

- Through hypnosis you can have even more control, because with hypnosis you suspend your usual mental limitations! Then you can use your imagination to rebuild yourself by under-limiting your limitations, as it were.

- Now I understand how the combination of hypnosis plus my unconscious mind can be used to improve my behaviour, and my emotional and physical well-being. Now I can see "the light at the end of the tunnel," and that light is GREEN!

So, Stan, you and I can plan, say, for the next week that we are going to have a "hell of a good time" every day! And even thinking that would change our genes.

- Over the next month, we could remember every positive, proud moment we've ever experienced in our whole lives. Our minds are going on *"search,"* and even though we don't know it, it'll continue searching for all those moments. We won't even know it, because the search is going on at our unconscious level. But remember, most of our life is lived on an unconscious level. Our conscious mind is just a tiny flashlight. It is very active, even when we don't know it!!!

- Researchers have conducted experiments where they flash photos of angry faces on the screen. People look at the screen, but they don't see the faces because they go by so quickly. When they measure the emotional response in the brain, it turns out the brain does notice. Amazing!!!

Psychotherapist:

The older I get, the more fascinated I am with the human mind and body. The whole notion of the unconscious mind which Freud really talked about many years ago is recently enjoying a resurgence with regard to Freud's contribution. Because the neuroscientists are finding out that the unconscious mind is doing a lot, like the experiment with the flashing faces, unconsciously we are picking things up.

Neuroscientists are in a way vindicating Freud's thesis that a lot of our activity is on an unconscious level. When you do hypnosis, you are kind of communicating with your own unconscious mind, which can be a mighty powerful friend, because it is full of creativity!!!

S*tan, these are the benefits of a positive outlook:*

- People with a more positive outlook on life—optimists— live longer than pessimists.
- People with a more positive outlook on life and its problems have lower incidences of heart diseases, including heart attacks.

- Optimistic people experience less pain and faster recovery times from illnesses and surgeries.

- We can increase our positive attitude by seeing negative experiences with some degree of positive outcome—in other words, hope!

- As I try to smile more, I feel more upbeat. People usually find smiles infectious. And so I receive a small reward by seeing my initial smile act as a catalyst for increasing, even to a small degree, the happiness of others.

- *PET, stands for Positron Emission Tomography. This scanning technique gives a three-dimension image of how body tissue, or an organ, is functioning, not just its structure. PET scans can show tumours, heart tissue, blood-flow, through the brain, et cetera. A short lived radioactive tracer is injected into the patient's bloodstream. After the radioactive tracer has circulated to the tissue of interest, the patient is placed into the PET imaging scanner.

Stan, because of my emotional condition, the following was given to me by a psychotherapist to become more motivated. It has been a big help to me so I thought I'd share it with you:

"The More things YOU DO,

Both Inside and Out,

The BETTER YOU Are

Going to FEEL."

by a psychotherapist

Chapter 17 – Thoughts regarding Time

The information below is taken from conversations with a psychotherapist.

Psychotherapist:

"Past": my memories of events that occurred before the *"present"*—that is, a former *"present"*.

"Present": when I experience awareness only in the immediate moment—that is, seeing a sunset, the smell of flowers, whatever happens from *"right now"* to *"right now"* to *"right now"* ... or what I experience every nanosecond between the past and the future.

"Future": what I imagine may happen later—that is, it will happen at a later *"present."*

Most people do not react in precisely the same way to the same situation or stimulus. For example, some past verbal abuses have caused deep corrosive perceptions of fear and shame in me. Other people would react to the same situations with similar (or, of course, different) response levels. Some of my experiences have resulted in lasting perceptions of extreme fear and shame.

Under *"Remembering,"* my described fearful/shameful feelings and pessimistic outlook, beginning from a very early age, became etched into or cemented onto my thoughts. However, although difficult, minimizing or eliminating my fears and shame is possible, because humans have the capacity to change attitudes! These are the steps which I am following to diminish my fears, shame, and depression, and to develop a more optimistic frame of mind, which requires continually choosing to change:

- When relating my past shame and fears to our support group, these etched-in painful memories slowly begin to change. They also change because I have already written these emotional wounds down on paper, which helps to get them out of my head. This is another step forward.

- For many years, I wasted energy by seeing and dwelling on my past negative feelings, failures, and regrets. Combined with observing these past thoughts, I also had a few worries about the future.

- I was stuck thinking about the past; it was like re-living the past in the "*present*" moment.

- My previous, almost inescapable, repeated painful thoughts of past emotional injuries, or "*looped thinking*," are diminishing, and are being replaced by a greater awareness of the "*present*."

Stan, here I go into a hypnotic trance regarding "the present", listening to the psychotherapist: for greater impact, I purposely changed the psychotherapist's "you" to "I" with his permission.

Psychotherapist:

Slowly, as I look back at my past, I am able to see my thoughts and feelings, not necessarily as "*being*" or "*feeling*" them. I have begun looking at my thoughts, and choosing not to identify them as my own feelings. Eventually, I have found some peace, and realized that I could only do that in the "*present*" moment. If I had kept thinking about the past I could not drop into that level of awareness of the "*present*."

On the other hand, if I were occupied in worrying about the future, I would not be able to drop into that state of awareness of the "*present*" moment. The only way I can find that peaceful state is to be in the "*present*" moment. By doing so, I find peace in the sense that I am aware of being aware of the "*present*," and that level of existence is timeless and peaceful and has no emotional suffering in it.

Now, more and more, I can look at my past negative thoughts and my negative feelings—without necessarily identifying myself with them.

As I learn to operate from a deeper level, a level of pure awareness of the "*present*," I spend a certain amount of my time in the "*present*" so that I can get down deep in just being aware—aware of the "*present*" moment.

I often tune out the frenetic worry about tomorrow, or regrets about yesterday and those of the distant past.

Now I have somewhat more energy to meet people. They pick up on my increasing peacefulness. They also pick up on the fact that I am actually listening to them—versus listening to me being only in the past, or into the future.

So, going back to the level of awareness is deeply connected to living in the "*present*," and to understand this is very, very critical!!!

So, when I write these painful feelings down, I feel that I can begin to forget them. And forgetting them has many good purposes. Forgetting means that the observations of the etched-in feelings become less distinct, and the cemented memories begin to crumble.

Another way is that I begin to think "*completely out of the box*," which is to say that I forgive family members with a sense of compassion and understanding, because their actions were coming from low self-esteem. And then I let go of these feelings. As the Buddhists say, "*I let go of the letting go*" and those feelings disappear into space, and get lost in time.

Yet another way is to realize that I am not those thoughts, I am not those feelings. As the Buddhists say, "*I can watch my feelings, and watch my thoughts and what am I watching?*" I am watching with "awareness" which is really who I am!!! Awareness in the "*present*"! When I limit awareness to the "*present*" time becomes timeless. The only time that we live in is the "*present*," even though we are able to think also in terms of the past and future. If I become stuck in thinking only of the past and future, I miss many experiences of the "*present*"!!!

Things take on a different perspective because I delve into the feeling of "*just being,*" knowing that I am not my thoughts, I am not my emotions—that is not what defines me. What does define me is simple "*consciousness*" or awareness of the "*present*"!!!

I can look upon shame and fear in a dispassionate way, and it does not touch "*my innermost being,*" which is really my "*true identity.*" It is a kind of "*being*" which I experience from time to time, "*when everything is clear, and I feel strong and solid in a way that is timeless.*"

Just enjoying the "*present*"—perhaps a colour, the sound of the wind in the trees, and I am totally in the "*present,*" and the past and the future disappear, and I learn to live in the "*present*" so the past is less and less relevant and I find peace, I find joy, and the simple awareness of myself as a being!!!

The freedom of just watching those thoughts and feelings of the past removed, that's the wisdom of many people, such as Buddha and Christ. Christ said, "*Look at the lilies of the field, they do not toil, they just are.*" And that feeling of just "*being*" is where my real identity lies, and it is not touched by my siblings, or by anyone else—it is my precious inner core. It is timeless, and comes alive when I find myself totally in the "*present*" because I am no longer a victim of time, or pain, or suffering of any kind!!!

I begin to realize that there is peace and just being aware without the usual harmful thoughts and feelings—pure auras, principles of peace, and joy.

In that awareness of "*the present*" I can enjoy the smell of fresh air and the sunrise in the morning.

I take particular interest in listening to melodies. Mozart wrote some incredibly beautiful music, mostly by instinct! Mozart was in touch with that deeper part of the self that just knew the notes to play in the "*present*" moment.

There are so many wonderful experiences that I am taking great joy in reading about and enjoying discovering that my wisdom begins to propel me into a different state of mind, it is full of the "*present moment.*"

S tan, *you can read much more on this topic in* "The Precious Present" *by Spencer Johnson, M.D., and* "The Power of Now" *by Eckhart Tolle.*

www.ingramcontent.com/pod-product-compliance
Lightning Source LLC
Chambersburg PA
CBHW051449170526
45166CB00001B/171